No Thanks, But Thanks!

... *for my food restrictions*

BRANDY GASSNER

No Thanks, But Thanks

Published by:
Professional Woman Publishing
www.pwnbooks.com

Cover photo credit:
Masinto/Dreamstime.com

ISBN: 978-0-9906109-9-1

Disclaimer

As much as I wish to help as many people as possible, and though I am a Certified Nutritional Consultant, I am not a doctor. Therefore, please do not use this book as a tool to diagnose yourself or your loved ones. Under no circumstances am I qualified to diagnose a disease or disorder, so please do not use the information in this book to do that. Nor am I qualified to tell you how to treat your disease/disorder. I am speaking from personal and professional experience, and the purpose of this book is to give you a reference guide to help you along your journey once you have spoken with the medical profession. This book is to be used in conjunction with your current treatment plan and to further your relationship with your team, not to replace it.

Dedication

Without my family, this book would never have come to fruition.

My kids have taught me so much over the years that there is no way I can say thank you adequately. I always thought that as a parent I was supposed to teach them – lesson number one learned. They have filled my life in a way that nobody but another parent could understand and I hope nothing but the best for the two lights in my life. I love you two more than anything.

My husband has never stood in the way of my dreams and has always supported me, even if he thought that particular dream was a little off the wall, and some were. But without his unwavering support and love, I would never have gotten to this point in my life. He works so hard to ensure that his whole family is safe, happy and loved - and for that I am truly blessed. It's not often you actually get the chance to marry your soul mate and grow more and more in love every day.

My parents, all three of them, have made me who I am. They always said, "Someday you will understand, and maybe even thank me". I understand, and thank you. Each one of you have your own way of getting through to me and have worked together to help me become the woman I hope you are proud to call your daughter.

My sister, aka best friend, has been there when it seemed like no one else was. From jumping in puddles as kids, to sitting in fields as women, she always made sure I made time for fun. Thank you for that – it is something I needed and didn't always know how to accomplish.

I wish words could express my love, appreciation, and gratitude to all of you.

Contents

Introduction

When my daughter was born in 2003 she was a sick young girl. It took us two years and a lot of grief to get a diagnosis for her. Once we got the diagnosis I was left in the dark. It took years of unnecessary pain and agony, physically and emotionally, to figure out what we were doing. No one told me what to do, how to do it, or how to find more information. Then we threw in our son to our familial mix who had his own set of health issues. We had a bit of an idea by then on how to manage, but we were still in the dark relatively speaking.

I looked everywhere for one book that would help me. One book that would tell me what I needed to know in simple language that my stressed out brain could comprehend. One book that told me that it would all work out. One book that I could reference for information, or at least tell me where to go for more information. One book I could loan to caregivers so they knew a bit about what was going on with my children. One book that I could keep track of all the information I needed. One book that would give me the confidence in myself to stand up to my doctors and tell them I thought they were wrong and needed to dig deeper for an answer. I never found it.

My goal is to compress years of experience into one handy reference guide for you. Whether you are the one who has been diagnosed with a disease or disorder that affects what you can eat or whether you have a loved one that you are concerned about. This book will serve as your one stop shop for definitions, explanations, notes, and inspiration.

There are thousands of books out there that can help you with Allergies, Diabetes, Celiac Disease, Gluten Intolerance, etc. They can help you with the nutrition part of it, the social aspect, or even help you understand the disease/disorder you have by reading through what other people have experienced. And they are all amazing books that can help you.

Why is this one different? This is different because I am not going to focus on just one disease/disorder. I am not going to write my own biography. I am not going to inundate you with complex medical terminology. I am going to make this short, sweet, easy to reference and useful for anyone who has to restrict the foods that they eat for whatever reason. I am going to throw in my personal and professional experience. I am going to leave you with hope, inspiration and a desire to learn more. I want to help you embrace this new life that has been diagnosed for you and not feel afraid, scared, intimidated or remorseful. Like I said to my friend as I started on my book writing journey, "It's amazing. Not only is there a light at the end of the tunnel, but there is this tunnel that I get to paint and create along the way!" I want you to feel the same way. Having a diagnosis is not a death sentence, it is a beginning; a starting point for you to discover new things and gain a further understanding into what makes your body tick.

This is a guide for you with quick to reference chapters, handy forms at the back of the book that you can copy and use as you need, or throw the book in your bag to carry with you and jot notes in as you think of them, with inspiration weaved through out it to keep you going on those days when you think, "I just can't take another day" or "does nobody understand and get it!?". Yes, you can take another day because you are the amazing you that has been given this challenge. I firmly believe we are only dealt what we can deal with, even though we may not understand it at the time. Someday we will. And someday, you will look back at this journey and actually appreciate it. It took years for me, but hopefully this book will shorten that time for you.

With love, health and hope,

Brandy

CHAPTER ONE

Defining Some Diseases and Disorders

I want to get the boring stuff out the way first. I want to explain what some of the diseases and/or disorders are that cause a person to restrict a type of food from their diet for whatever reason. My main goal is to provide brief, yet concise information for you that you can easily reference. I will have to throw in some fancy terminology for you, but I will try to keep it to a minimum. If you want more information on each disease/disorder, I have provided a list of resources in the last chapter that are reputable and full of information for you.

This is intended to be a quick, easy to reference guide to get you started. Who knows, maybe one day I will write books on individual diseases to get into the nitty gritty and provide recipes specifically for each restrictive diet... but for now, I just want to provide everyone with an overview so that a basic understanding can be achieved and a journey can be embraced.

Celiac Disease

DEFINITION: Celiac Disease is an autoimmune disorder that is genetically linked and can affect people at any age. People with Celiac Disease have an immune response to eating certain grains that contain gluten that causes the villi in their small intestine to flatten out, in turn losing the ability to absorb nutrients, leading to malnutrition and a host of other complications depending on the severity. Celiac is not an allergy, nor is it an intolerance. This disease causes internal damage that is responsible for a wide range of complications.

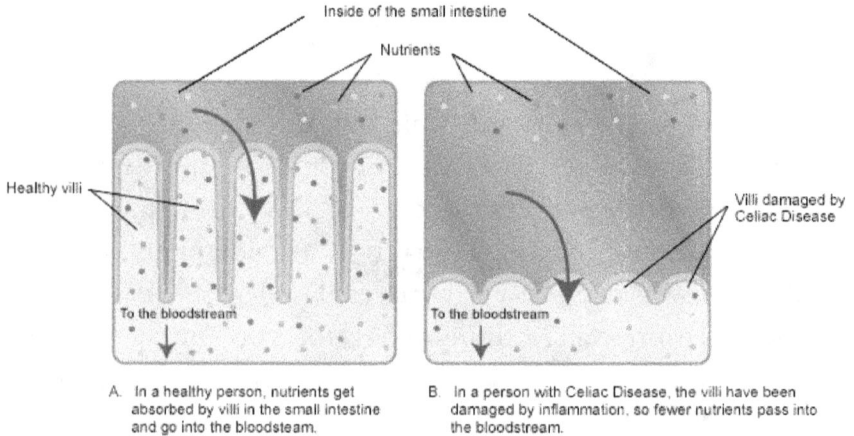

Inside of the small intestine

Nutrients

Healthy villi

Villi damaged by Celiac Disease

To the bloodstream

To the bloodstream

A. In a healthy person, nutrients get absorbed by villi in the small intestine and go into the bloodsteam.

B. In a person with Celiac Disease, the villi have been damaged by inflammation, so fewer nutrients pass into the bloodstream.

© Children's Hospital Boston 2009

(2)

The grains that contain gluten (the protein found in the endosperm of certain grains) are wheat, barley and rye as well as their related grains (bulgar, couscous, durum, kamut, etc). Pure oats do not contain gluten, but because oats are often processed on the same equipment as the other grains, the potential of cross contamination is very real. If you are going to eat oats, ensure that they are pure oats and are labelled "gluten free". It is recommended that you should avoid oats for at least the first year of being diagnosed and then carefully try them if you choose to at a later date.

SYMPTOMS: The symptoms of this disease vary depending on the age of the patient. Many of the symptoms are also confused with other disorders such as lactose intolerance or irritable bowel syndrome. Different people may show different symptoms because they may be in a different stage of diagnosis (they may have just developed the disease and are just beginning to show signs, or they may have had the disease for years and are showing another set of symptoms that are because of malnourishment). Symptoms are also relevant to the amount of gluten that has been consumed to date. Here is a sampling of some of the symptoms that are shown at various ages.

Children

- Growth problems
- Vomiting
- Irritability
- Fatigue
- Chronic diarrhea, with or without blood
- Decreased appetite
- Failure to gain weight
- Abdominal bloating and pain

Teens

- Disease is often triggered by a stressful situation such as leaving for college, injury, illness, or pregnancy
- Delayed puberty
- Diarrhea
- Depression
- Weight loss
- Eczema
- Abdominal pain and bloating
- Growth problems
- Mouth sores

Adults

- Osteoporosis due to inability to absorb calcium
- Bone and joint pain
- Irregular menstrual periods
- Seizures
- Depression or anxiety
- Arthritis
- Anemia due to iron deficiency
- Infertility and/or miscarriages
- Tingling and/or numbness in hands and feet

TREATMENT: Treatment is strict avoidance of any food that contains gluten. This is getting easier and easier as more companies are producing gluten free foods. The reason strict avoidance is required is multifaceted. First of all, you will feel much better. Secondly, you will be reducing your risk of malnutrition and the problems that come with that, liver diseases and cancer of the intestine. Hair loss and dental problems in kids that continue it ingest gluten are common, and can be completely avoided by adopting a gluten free diet.

Crohn's /Colitis

DEFINITION: Crohn's disease is characterized by inflammation in the intestines. It mainly causes ulcerations, or breaks in the lining, of the small and large intestine but can affect any part of the digestive system from the mouth to the bottom end. The only difference between this and Colitis (or Ulcerative Colitis) is where the inflammation is occurring. In Colitis, only the colon is involved. Quite often these two diseases are talked about at the same time using the term *Inflammatory Bowel Disease.*

Inflammatory Bowel Disease

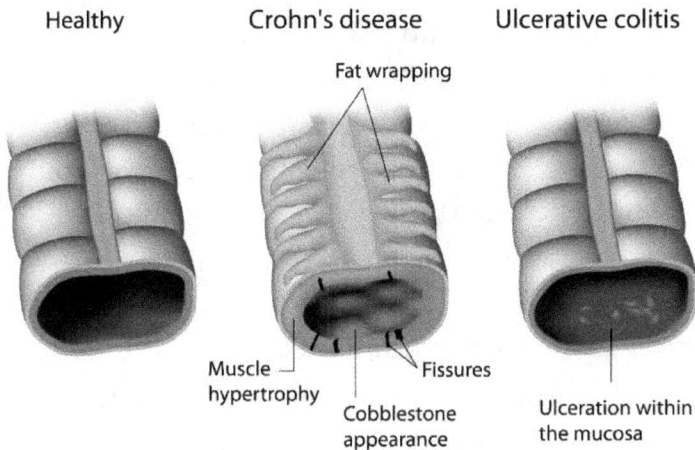

Healthy   Crohn's disease   Ulcerative colitis

Fat wrapping

Muscle hypertrophy   Fissures

Cobblestone appearance

Ulceration within the mucosa

(4)

In early stages of Crohn's small erosions form on the inner surface of the bowel, then as the disease progresses, the erosions become deeper and larger forming true ulcers that will scar and cause the bowel to become stiffer. Further into the progression, the bowel becomes more narrowed, less motile, and ultimately can become constricted. As the ulcers grow and puncture holes through the wall of the bowel, the bacteria from the bowel can spread to adjacent organs and cause infection.

SYMPTOMS – CROHN'S: Symptoms vary depending on whether there is an obstruction or an ulcer. If you have an obstruction, which is most likely to occur in the small intestine rather than the colon, the symptoms are:

- Severe abdominal cramps
- Diarrhea
- Vomiting
- Nausea
- Weight loss
- Distention (bloating)

If your symptoms are caused by ulcers you may experience:

- Abdominal abscess (if the ulcer reaches through to an empty space, a collection of infected pus will form) causing tender masses, high fever, and abdominal pain.
- Fistulas (when the ulcer goes through to an adjacent organ) cause various symptoms depending on which organ they are formed between
  - Enteric-vesicular (fistula between the intestine and bladder) cause urinary tract infections, and passing of gas and feces during urination
  - Enteric-cutaneous (fistula between intestine and skin) cause mucous and pus to form a small sore on the skin of the abdomen – quite painful
  - Colonic-vaginal (fistula between the colon and vagina) causes gas and fecal matter to pass through the vagina
  - Anal fistulas form from the intestines to the anus and cause mucous and pus to emerge from the fistula's opening around the anus.

SYMPTOMS – COLITIS: For people who suffer from Colitis, their symptoms are generally restricted to the large colon, therefore their symptoms are:

- Diarrhea
- Rectal bleeding
- Gas/bloating
- Abdominal pain

Depending on what area of the colon and the extent of damage that is caused, Colitis can be further broken down into these categories with the associated symptoms:

- Ulcerative proctitis has inflammation limited to the rectum so mild intermittent bleeding may be the only symptom expressed, sometimes along with rectal pain, urgency, and an ineffective painful urge to go.

- Proctosigmoiditis indicates inflammation of the rectum and sigmoid colon (area of the colon that is closest to the rectum). Symptoms are the same as above as well as cramping and bloody diarrhea.

- Left-sided colitis is just as it sounds; it is inflammation that goes from the rectum up the left side of the colon and includes cramping, weight loss, left side abdominal pain and bloody diarrhea as symptoms.

- Pancolitis is a term used to describe inflammation of the whole colon. Sometimes, the general term of colitis is used for this. The whole colon includes the right side, left side, transverse colon, and the rectum therefore symptoms are much more varied. They include abdominal pain, fever, night sweats, cramping, and bloody diarrhea. This is the worst case scenario of symptoms. If the inflammation is mild, then symptoms are less severe. Often people with Pancolitis suffer from other diseases as well and there is a whole symphony of symptoms that are sometimes related to colitis or mistakenly attributed to the colitis.

- Fulminant colitis is a rare form of Pancolitis and is much more severe. These people are extremely ill and suffer symptoms such as dehydration, incomprehensible abdominal pain, and chronic diarrhea with bleeding and sometimes even shock. Often hospitalization is required for this form of diarrhea and medication and sometimes surgery is required to ease symptoms.

As for both Crohn's and Colitis, because the inflammation comes and goes, regardless of where the inflammation is, the symptoms will come and go for each individual. Sometimes the symptoms will be unbearable, other times they are a mild annoyance. Because of the irregularity (pardon the pun) of the inflammation, these two diseases are quite distressing and can be embarrassing. Treatment is important to maintain, even if you are without symptoms, to help maintain a balance of normalcy.

TREATMENT: Treatment for these two diseases are directly related to the location, severity and associated complications. If your symptoms are mild you may not need treatment, same as if you are in remission. There is no cure for Crohn's or Colitis so the goals of treatment are to encourage remission, maintain remission, to improve quality of life and to offset the side effects of any medication that may be needed.

Different types of medication may work for these diseases, and often doctors will need to try you on different types to see which one works best for you with the least amount of side effects. They also want to use as low as dosage as possible to further reduce any side effects. This will take some patience on your part because it is a trial and error process.

If surgery is recommended for severe cases, it is generally not to get rid of Crohn's or Colitis, it is to remove the part of the intestine that is causing an obstruction or infection, drain pus or abscesses from the abdomen or rectum, or to treat severe anal fistulae that do not respond to pharmacological treatment. Another reason for surgery, particularly for Colitis patients, is to remove parts of the colon where the lining has changed in a way to increase the risk for colon cancer.

From a dietary perspective, there are a few options people with Crohn's or Colitis can do to help ease their symptoms. First of all, if you are having a flare up, eating very soft foods can help, even going as far as pureeing your foods in a blender. The reasoning behind this is simple – the softer your foods, the easier your intestines have to work to pass the food through. For severe Crohn's symptoms a total liquid diet may help, or even intravenous nutrition may be recommended. Also, insoluble fibre is hard to digest, so keeping that fibre level on the lower side is often recommended. Also, because the intestines need to heal, good quality sources of protein are suggested to help the tissues heal. Primarily though, it is important to eat a balanced nutrition diet that is tolerable to you at the point you are at.

Another aspect of treatment that can help some people are anti-diarrhea medications such as Imodium®, Pepto-Bismol®, etc. This will help with the cramping, diarrhea and may help with the feeling of urgency long enough to get you to a bathroom in time.

Diabetes

DEFINITION: Diabetes is categorized as one of three types; Type 1 Diabetes (formally known as Juvenile Diabetes) is often diagnosed in children and adolescents and is diagnosed when the pancreas is not able to produce insulin. Type 2 Diabetes is diagnosed when the pancreas does not produce enough insulin or when the body is not able to use that insulin as well as it should. The final type of Diabetes is call Gestational Diabetes and is a temporary condition that happens to pregnant women. It often goes away after child birth, but it does increase the risk for mother and child to develop Diabetes.

Insulin is a hormone that regulates glucose in the blood. Glucose is one of the main sources of energy for our body and is obtained by breaking down carbohydrates such as pasta, rice, bread, etc and obviously from sugary food sources such as sweets, pop, etc. When a person eats food and their glucose levels rise in response, their pancreas reacts by producing and releasing insulin to pick up that glucose in the blood. Because the insulin is either lacking or not used properly in people with Diabetes, their cells are not able to pick up glucose from the bloodstream efficiently. Therefore too much glucose is left in the bloodstream causing an array of symptoms.

TYPE 1 DIABETES		TYPE 2 DIABETES
3 million Americans have it	**#**	22 million Americans have it
Usually appears before age 40	**age**	Generally appears after age 40
Body doesn't produce insulin	**insulin**	Body produces insulin, it doesn't work efficiently
Unknown, but likely linked to environmental/genetic triggers	**cause**	Family history, poor diet, low activity level and obesity increase risk
People with Type 1 take insulin shots	**treatment**	Oral medication, lifestyle changes, sometimes treated with insulin

(3)

SYMPTOMS: As with any condition the symptoms depend on the severity of the disease. Generally speaking, Type 1 Diabetes symptoms come on suddenly whereas the symptoms come on more gradual with Type 2 Diabetes. Some of the most common symptoms of Diabetes are:

- Unusual thirst
- Slow healing cuts/bruises
- Weight change (either gain or loss)
- Frequent urination
- Blurry vision
- Extreme fatigue or lack of energy
- Tingling/numbness in hands or feet
- Dry itchy skin

TREATMENT: Treatment for Diabetes depends on whether you have Type 1, Type 2, or Gestational Diabetes. Nutrition is extremely important in managing your Diabetes. What you eat, when you eat, and how much you eat, all play an important part in your blood glucose levels. This is when having a nutritionist or dietician work with you is important because he/she will be able to educate you on your diet.

Sometimes if you have Type 2 Diabetes you can manage it adequately with diet and exercise. Other times you may need to use insulin injections and/or other medication as well. Type 1 Diabetics always need to use insulin injections and sometimes medication as well. This is when glucose testing and working closely with your medical team are critical. Your glucose levels decide how much insulin you need to take. Accuracy, consistency, and honesty with yourself are incredibly important when working with your medication.

Important parts of Diabetes are learning about the Glycemic Index (GI) or Glycemic Load (GL) of foods and learn how to eat using this invaluable tool. I have included a few links in chapter 9 to help you start learning about this, as well as put in a short chart in the appendix to help you.

Basically, the Glycemic Index (GI) is a way to rank your carbohydrates on a scale from 0 – 100 based on how much they raise your blood glucose levels after eating. Low GI foods gradually increase your blood glucose levels, whereas the higher the food is on the GI scale, the faster that food will raise your blood glucose levels. The Glycemic Load (GL) takes this concept one step further by also factoring in the amount of food that is ingested.

The basic goal is when working with the Glycemic Index is to choose foods that are 55 or less most often, moderately choose foods between 56 and 69, and try to steer clear of foods ranked 70 or higher. If you do choose higher GI foods, try to pair them with very low GI foods. When using the Glycemic Load, the goal is the same, choose from low GL foods (ranking of 0 – 10), moderately from the middle (11 – 19) and rarely from the high (20 +).

I am not going to get into too much detail in this book about working with the Glycemic Index or Glycemic Load of foods. There are whole books dedicated to that, and one in my future plans. But for now, try to educate yourself as much as possible by using the resources I have provided as well as what your dietician/nutritionist/doctor have given you.

Diverticulitis

DEFINITION: Diverticulitis is a disorder where pouches form along the wall of the intestine and get inflamed or infected. Generally they form along the colon, but they can be located anywhere along the intestinal tract. This inflammation/infection can be very painful and is caused when fecal matter gets trapped in the small pouches allowing bacteria to grow.

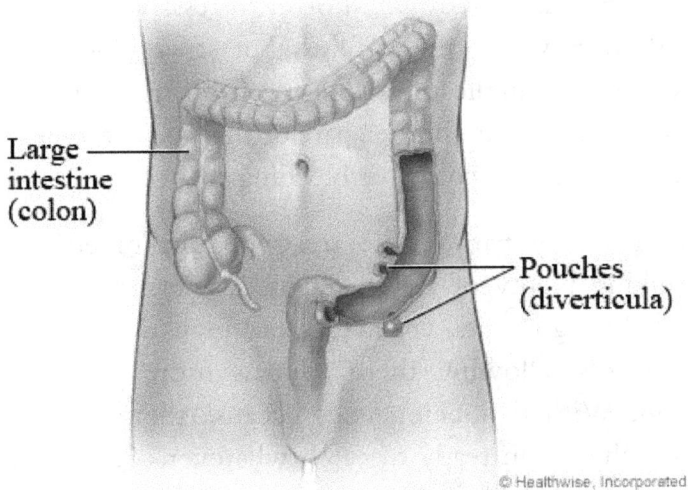

Large intestine (colon)

Pouches (diverticula)

© Healthwise, Incorporated

(5)

SYMPTOMS: Generally symptoms last from a few hours to a few weeks, depending on the severity of the infection that is present. The most common symptoms are:

- Belly pain in the lower left side that worsens when you move
- Fever and chills
- Loss of appetite
- Cramps
- Nausea/vomiting
- Bloating/gas
- Periods of constipation then diarrhea

TREATMENT: Treatment, again, depends on the severity of the symptoms. If you are only suffering from cramps, gas, and abdominal pain, then using a heating pad, relaxing and taking an over the counter pain killer may help. Other times, you may need to take antibiotics to help with the infection and go on a clear liquid diet until the pain goes away. For the most severe cases, you may be admitted to the hospital for IV medication and nutrition to allow the bowel to rest. Very few people ever need surgery for diverticulitis, but if you do, it is generally because of complication resulting from it, such as an infection that has spread to another part of the body, a blocked colon, a narrowing of the colon, or bleeding that cannot be stopped.

Again, a key part of the treatment for diverticulitis is diet. Drinking plenty of water, gradually increasing the amount of fibre through fruits, vegetables and brans will help add bulk to the stools, allowing them to pass more easily through the colon. With that being said, because there are little pouches along the colon ready to catch whatever comes their way, it is recommended to avoid nuts and seeds that can easily get trapped in there. Nutritionally speaking, the nutrition that nuts and seeds provide you can be easily replaced. Where the trick comes in is realizing all the nuts and seeds that are out there that you eat without realizing it! Think about all those little seeds on a strawberry...

Eosinophilic Gastrointestinal Disorders

DEFINITION: Eosinophilic Gastrointestinal Disorders are characterized by having an increased amount of eosinophils, a type of white blood cell, in a particular location(s) of the gastrointestinal tract, from the esophagus all the way through. Depending on where the eosinophil count is high causing the inflammation, is how they decide to classify it. The different classifications are:

- Eosinophilic Esophagitis – high number of eosinophils in the esophagus; this is the most common of all Eosinophilic Disorders, therefore it is the most researched

- Eosinophilic Gastritis – high number of eosinophils in the stomach
- Eosinophilic Gastroenteritis – high number of eosinophils in multiple parts of the gastrointestinal tract
- Eosinophilic Colitis – high number of eosinophils in the large intestine

One of the challenges in diagnosing Eosinophilic Disorders is that there is not a standardized diagnostic criterion for them, other than for Eosinophilic Esophagitis, which is the most common form of Eosinophilic Disorder. And even then, the physician needs to look at both the pathology and symptoms and then rule out other medical issues that may be causing the symptoms, such as reflux. The one thing that can be agreed on when diagnosing a person with an Eosinophilic Disorder, is that a scope needs to be performed, with multiple biopsies taken, to look at the number of eosinophils in the affected area and the damage and/or inflammation that is present. The biopsies must be taken because the affected area can look perfectly normal, it is the biopsies that tell the story.

Eosinophilic Disorders are also closely tied with allergies and asthma. This disorder has been called "the mother of all food allergies" because a person may be severely restricted in the foods that they can eat. Quite often a person with this type of disorder is also allergic to one or more foods, which trigger a reaction in the gastrointestinal tract. The person's body sees the molecular food protein as an "invader" and attacks it by sending out eosinophils to quash it. Environmental factors can even aggravate the symptoms. And the intriguing part of the equation is that eosinophils are also the same cell that cause inflammation in the lungs associated with asthma. In my own personal experience, I have found that when a person with this disorder suffers an asthma attack, often their Eosinophilic Disorder will flare as well.

SYMPTOMS: Symptoms vary immensely for this group of disorders, depending on severity, age, and location. Here is a brief overview of the symptoms that may arise for each classification of Eosinophilic Disorder:

- Eosinophilic Esophagitis – common to all ages
    - Dysphasia – difficulty swallowing
    - Food getting stuck in esophagus
    - Chest pain
    - Abdominal pain
    - Difficulty sleeping
    - Reflux that does not respond to medication
    - Nausea
    - Vomiting

- Eosinophilic Esophagitis – infants/children
    - Failure to thrive
    - Poor appetite, food refusal

- Symptoms of other Eosinophilic Disorders vary depending on where the inflammation is, how long it has been there, and to a degree the age of the patient. In addition to the symptoms above, the person may also experience:
    - Malnutrition
    - Anemia
    - Blood in the stool
    - Diarrhea
    - Delayed emptying of the stomach
    - Bloating

Table 2. Clinical Symptoms of Eosinophilic Esophagitis

Symptom	Range (%)
CHILDREN	
Heartburn/regurgitation	5-82
Emesis	8-100
Abdominal pain	5-68
Dysphagia	16-100
Food impaction	10-50
Failure to thrive	5-19
Chest pain	17-20
Diarrhea	1-24
Other[a]	Not reported
ADULTS	
Intermittent dysphagia	29-100
Food impaction	25-100
Heartburn/regurgitation	7-100
Chest pain	1-58
Abdominal pain	3-25
Other[b]	Not reported

[a] *Nausea, respiratory symptoms (cough, wheezing, sinusitis), choking, pneumonia, aversive feeding behavior, and slow growth.*
[b] *Diarrhea and weight loss were reported in some patients, with many patients experiencing repeated food impactions prior to diagnosis.*
Source: *References 1, 2.*

(6)

TREATMENT: The treatment for Eosinophilic Disorders is extremely variable depending on symptoms, severity, location, physician, and associated medical problems. In my research I have also discovered that different countries have different approaches to treatment. Depending on what you and your physician agree on, you will have to work closely with a whole team to figure out what works best for you. Some physicians may try medication first to see if that works, in addition to elimination diets; others may go directly to tube feeding cutting out all foods and trying to add in foods one at a time to see what will work.

Because Eosinophilic Disorders are so closely related to food allergies, quite often a visit to the allergist for allergy testing is recommended. If there are any food allergies detected, then the avoidance of those are to be adhered to. Sometimes this is all it takes for symptoms to be resolved. Other times, using a medication to keep inflammation down can be used, such as swallowing the same medication used to be inhaled for asthma maintenance, or a corticosteroid over a period of time to take down the inflammation. Other times, you need to play with your diet to see what foods are triggering your symptoms. This is done by removing a certain food, usually starting with your common top eight allergy foods, then reintroducing them to see if any symptoms return. In the more extreme cases, an elemental diet is required. That is when the person receives most, or all, of their nutrition through a specialized formula that is also used to tube feed people. This type of formula has no whole protein in it for the person's body to react to, therefore it is safe. Some people take enough of this orally, while others require gastric tubes to maintain their nutritional status.

Depending on your doctor, they may rely on you to introduce a food and wait for symptoms or they may want to introduce one or two foods for a couple weeks/months, and then repeat a scope to do a biopsy to count the eosinophils. This is where your physicians' preference and practice comes into play. Other physicians only scope when the symptoms are not manageable.

Food Allergies

DEFINITION: Food allergies are defined as hypersensitivity disorder of the immune system. Your body mistakenly interprets food protein (on a molecular level) as harmful and are tagged by immunoglobulin E (IgE) triggering your body to react as if there was an invader in your body. Obviously, your body is going to do it's best to get rid of that invader, and it does so by sending out white blood cells to attack- causing the allergic reaction. Basically, it is your body's way of saying, "Hey! I don't like that so I am going to give you this reaction so you stop feeding me this food" which for many other people they can eat without a problem. In a true allergic reaction, your body will react within seconds to hours of ingesting the problematic food.

Eight foods are responsible for 90% of the food allergies out there. They are:

- Cow's milk
- Eggs
- Fish
- Peanuts
- Shellfish
- Soy
- Tree nuts
- Wheat

SYMPTOMS: Reactions range from mild discomfort, to anaphylaxis (which is a life threatening reaction causing swelling in the airways, tingling in the mouth, scalp, feet or hands, and/or trouble breathing). Some of the most common symptoms are:

- Hives or red, itchy skin
- Stuffy or itchy nose, sneezing or itchy, teary eyes
- Vomiting, stomach cramps or diarrhea
- Angioedema or swelling

SKIN	RESPIRATORY	GASTROINTESTINAL	CARDIOVASCULAR	NEUROLOGICAL
hives, swelling, itching, warmth, redness	coughing, wheezing, shortness of breath, chest pain or tightness, throat tightness, trouble swallowing, hoarse voice, nasal congestion or hay fever-like symptoms, (sneezing or runny or itchy nose; red, itchy or watery eyes)	nausea, stomach pain or cramps, vomiting, diarrhea	dizziness/ lightheadedness, pale/blue colour, weak pulse, fainting, shock, loss of consciousness	anxiety, feeling of "impending doom" (feeling that something really bad is about to happen), headache
				OTHER[23]
				uterine cramps

(7)

TREATMENT: Treatment varies, depending on the severity of the reaction. Most often, people will use an antihistamine to help with the hives, rash, etc. when they come in contact with an allergen. Depending on the severity, and epinephrine auto injector (EpiPen®, Twinject®, or Allerject®) may be required. The best way to treat a food allergy is through avoidance. If you don't ingest the food, you can't have a reaction. Unfortunately, that chocolate on the table is just too irresistible for some, and knowingly, they will chance the reaction for that one taste. The tricky thing with food allergies is though, that the more the body is exposed to the allergen, the quicker and more severe the reaction is. So, yes, that one bite of chocolate didn't bother you too bad last time, but if you have a clinical allergy to it, then this might be the time when the hives are so bad that you need to go to the emergency room. Taking a chance with food allergies is like playing Russian Roulette – you never know how severe the next reaction will be.

Food Intolerance

DEFINITION: Food Intolerance is where you are not able to eat a food because it causes symptoms without the physiological IgE response. Food intolerances are not life threatening, whereas true allergies can be potentially life threatening. Food intolerance symptoms usually comes on gradually, may only happen if you eat too much of a certain food or consume the food too often. Intolerances are your body's way of saying, "I'm not too happy with eating this, so please stop now before I give you even more gas."

To determine if the symptoms you are experiencing are an intolerance or clinical allergy, you will need to see an allergist so that they can perform allergy tests. These tests will determine if they are true IgE allergies, or an intolerance.

The main difference between allergy and intolerance is that histamine and immunoglobulin E (IgE) are part of the physiological allergic response, whereas with intolerances the individual only suffers from the same symptoms without the clinical response in intolerant reactions. Because of the body's reaction to food protein (on a molecular level, not the protein we think of when we think of meat, beans, and nuts), if you have true clinical allergies that have an increase in IgE when the body reacts to it, the chances for anaphylaxis is there.

Intolerances can be a result of missing enzymes needed to digest a food, or a result of the body's inability to absorb nutrients from the food. An example of a missing enzyme causing a food intolerance is lactose intolerance. When a person is lactose intolerant, they are missing the enzyme lactase that is required to digest lactose properly. Thankfully, there are lactase tablets you can take prior to ingesting lactose that can help your body digest the lactose. Alternatively, there are even lactose free products out there (not dairy free, but lactose free) that you can purchase and enjoy freely.

SYMPTOMS: Some symptoms of food intolerance can be the same as allergy such as:

- nausea
- vomiting
- diarrhea
- stomach pain

Other symptoms that are just due to intolerance are

- gas
- cramps
- bloating
- heartburn
- headaches
- irritability (who wouldn't be cranky if they were feeling rotten!)

With intolerances, you do not get the rashes, hives, itchy skin, breathing problems, chest pain, or anaphylactic symptoms.

TREATMENT: Treatment for food intolerance varies, depending on the food and the severity. You may need to either avoid the food completely or just cut back on it. If you are lactose intolerant, you can drink lactose free milk, or take a lactase enzyme before consuming cow's milk to help your body digest the lactose. If you are intolerance to wheat, you may not be able to eat a whole sandwich, but having a cracker now and then probably won't hurt you. The positive spin to having a food intolerance is you know ingesting the food won't kill you and that there is no physical damage being done to your insides, like with Celiac Disease.

Irritable Bowel Syndrome

DEFINITION: Irritable Bowel Syndrome is a difficult thing to pin down. Some people swear that it is its own disorder; other people have the opinion that it is a term created to explain the pain people have when there is no other explanation that they can figure out for it. Regardless of mine or your opinion of it, IBS is diagnosed in approximately 10% to 20% of the population of the Western world. So it is very real, and relatively common.

IBS is defined as a chronic condition of the lower gastrointestinal tract that causes a variety of symptoms and based on the most common symptom, patients can fall into one of four categories:

- Diarrhea and Pain
- Diarrhea, Constipation and Pain
- Constipation and Pain
- Unsubtyped

IBS does not lead to more serious diseases like Crohn's or Cancer. Nor is it an inflammatory condition that can cause permanent damage to your intestine. What it is, is a disorder that comes and goes and is associated with stress levels. It can be debilitating for many people, or just a simple annoyance with the odd cramp here and there. It is theorized that people with IBS have irregular contractions in their bowel. Sometimes, they have only 6 peristaltic contractions per hour, while other times they may have upwards of 25 or 30! No wonder people with IBS get cramps and feel uncomfortable – their bowels never know what is coming next.

The cause of IBS is not well understood and still being researched. But a general consensus is that there is a combination of physical and mental issues that lead to IBS. Those issues are:

- Signals between the brain and nerves of the intestines are not getting through correctly

- Motility, or movement, of the colon is irregular

- People with IBS have a lower pain tolerance for bowel stretching than other people so the brain processes the pain differently compared to people without IBS

- Stress, anxiety, depression, and other psychological issues are common in people with IBS and can exacerbate symptoms

- Some people who have had a bacterial infection or too much "friendly" bacteria in the gut, can develop IBS

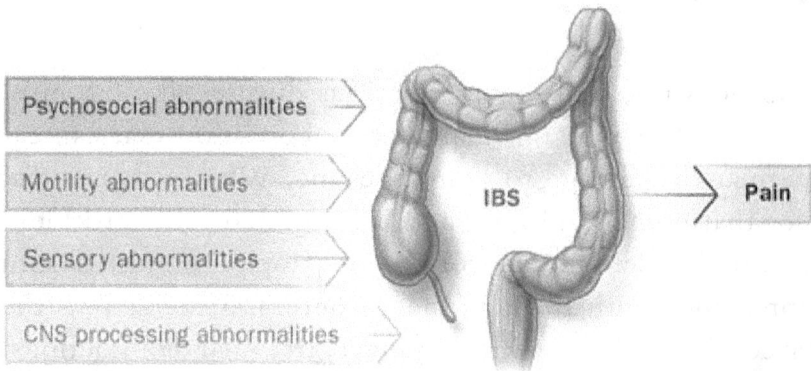

Psychosocial abnormalities

Motility abnormalities

Sensory abnormalities

CNS processing abnormalities

IBS

Pain

(8)

SYMPTOMS: Symptoms of IBS are varied, depending on the person. In order to receive a diagnosis of IBS, abdominal pain or discomfort needs to be associated with at least two of the following associated symptoms:

- Bowel movements that produce a relief from the abdominal discomfort that was previously felt
- Stools that are different than normal, either more watery or harder and lumpier than usual
- A change in the frequency of bowel movements, whether it is more frequent or less often

Other symptoms that can go along with IBS are:

- Bloating
- Mucus in the stool
- Headaches
- Urgency to go with no effectiveness
- Feeling that the bowel movement has not been completed
- Nausea
- Early satiety (feeling full early)
- Heartburn
- Fatigue
- Lower back pain

It is important to remember, that because IBS is multifaceted, some of these symptoms may be more directly related to another issue other than the IBS. For example, many people who have IBS also physically react more to stress than other people. So, that headache may be more attributable to stress levels than IBS.

TREATMENT: Treating IBS can be tricky because there is no known cause for it, so researchers are unable to pinpoint exactly what needs to be treated. Therefore, most treatment plans are geared toward relieving the symptoms for each person based on an individual basis. Most often, symptoms can be treated by a few lifestyle changes. Sometimes, for the more severe cases, medication can be prescribed. If you suffer from diarrhea primarily, there are medications that will relax the colon and slow down the movement of stool through your intestinal tract. If you suffer from the constipation type, then there are medications that can draw fluid into the intestine to help soften the stool. You can also get similar products over the counter, but if they are severe, then your doctor may decide to prescribe you these type of drugs.

Other prescription drugs that your doctor and you may decide are beneficial can include antidepressants to either a) help with depression if that is one of your coinciding factors, or b) help inhibit the neurons (brain cells) that control the intestines. One aspect of antidepressants that most people don't always understand, is that they have other uses in addition to treating depression, so if your doctor suggests using them, it is not always because he thinks you are depressed. There are other clinical uses for them.

Other treatment options for IBS that you can follow are:

- Fibre supplements for constipation
- Ant–diarrhea medications
- Avoiding or limiting foods that create a lots of gas if you suffer from bloating (cabbage, beans, broccoli, soft drinks, etc)
- Learning what foods trigger your IBS. For some people, coffee, milk, wheat, alcohol, sweeteners, and very high fibre foods trigger their symptoms. The best way to figure this out is to keep track of what you eat and what your symptoms are. Check the appendix for a form to help you with this.

PKU (Phenylketonuria)

DEFINITION: PKU is a rare disease where people are unable to process the amino acid phenylalanine (the *Phenyl* in Phenylketonuria) because they lack an enzyme that completes the process. I hate to do this to you, but I am going to have to get into some biology to explain how this disease works.

When we eat food and it goes through the process of digestion, first thing that happens is we mechanically break down the food by chewing it and mixing it with our saliva. Then, our stomach acids further break it down. Once that happens, our body breaks the nutrient molecules further into amino acids using enzymes. Different enzymes are required to break down different molecules. For example, the enzyme lactase is used to break down the bonds in lactose, the sugar found in milk; diastase breaks down vegetable starch; and lipase helps break down fats found in dairy, oils, nuts and meats.

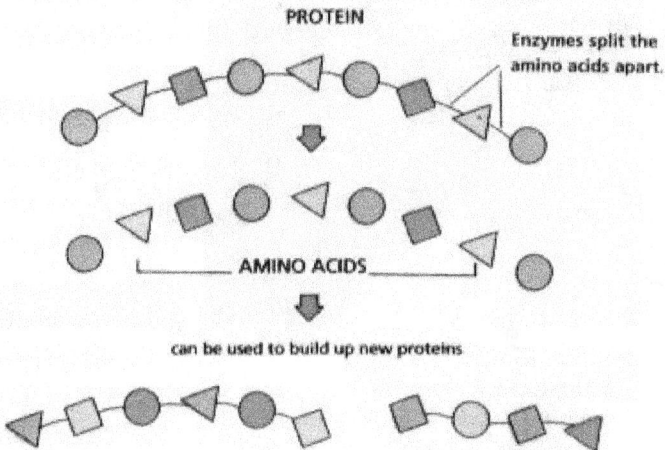

PROTEIN

Enzymes split the amino acids apart.

AMINO ACIDS

can be used to build up new proteins

(9)

31

The reason enzymes break down protein molecules down is to create amino acids, which are used to build new proteins that our body needs for growth, metabolism, moving nutrients and oxygen in our body, etc. The way amino acids are put together to build new proteins is through enzymes as well.

The enzyme phenyl-alanine hydroxylase is used with the amino acid phenylalanine to construct new proteins. People who have PKU do not have the enzyme phenyl-alanine hydroxylase. Therefore, they are unable use the phenylalanine amino acid to build new proteins. That causes a build up of phenylalanine in the body. Confused yet?

All you really need to know is that this is a genetic disorder that is life long, has no cure, and does not allow the person the innate ability to build the necessary proteins for normal development. But it is rather to nice to know why isn't it?

SYMPTOMS: The symptoms of PKU are as follows:

- Lighter skin or hair (phenylalanine is responsible for building the proteins for the pigment for hair and skin color)
- Delayed mental and social skills
- Below normal head size
- Tremors
- Skin rashes
- Jerky movements of legs/arms
- Hyperactivity
- Intellectual disabilities
- Feeling of anxiety or depression
- Irritability
- A musty odor on breath or skin or in urine (this is a direct result of the build up of phenylalanine)

TREATMENT: Treatment for PKU is to follow a diet that is low in phenylalanine, especially during the developmental years. If you do not ingest the amino acid, then it cannot accumulate in your system. Often, a formula called Lofenalac®, is used as a protein source to ensure that the other proteins that can be ingested are being taken in, allowing for adequate growth and development. As with Eosinophilic Disorders, this formula is the main source of nutrition, and it is supplemented with food.

Because that particular amino acid is related to brain development, taking fish oil supplements to replace the fatty acids missing from the phenylalanine free diet, may help with brain development and co-ordination. Working closely with a dietician is important because close monitoring of your diet will need to be done to ensure that you are not also missing other important vitamins and minerals due to the food restrictions.

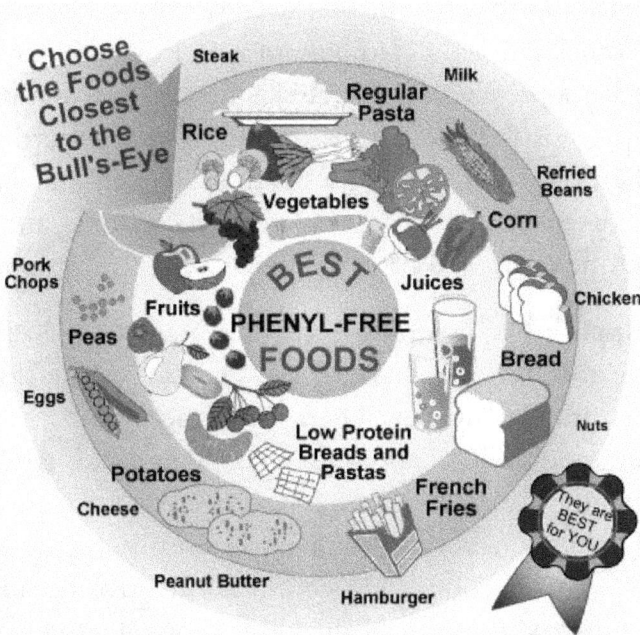

(10)

Summary

Hopefully, I have left you with a little bit of an understanding of what some of the diseases/disorders are that cause a person to restrict certain foods from their diet for whatever reason. Of course, not every possible disease/disorder has been covered. But I have covered some of the more common ones that you may come across and given you a bit of a start on understanding what you or a loved one may be up against. Of course, this is just a teaser in regards to the information that is available to you. I urge you to look in the last chapter for a list of reputable places to go for more information.

If after reading this you think to yourself, "Hey! That sounds just like me (or your loved one) and what I am going through," be careful not to jump the gun and self diagnose yourself. I know that the information available to you via the internet, this book, other books, friends, family, etc is immense and we can learn an incredible amount from these resources. But, it takes a professional to actually do the tests and provide a clinical diagnosis. You can arm yourself with information so that when you do go to visit the doctor you have the knowledge and tools to discuss your symptoms, ask knowledgeable questions, and have a productive conversation.

For example, if after doing some research, and deciding on your own that you may have Celiac Disease, you decide to cut out gluten from your diet. Then when the time comes for the physician to do the scope and take biopsies to confirm the diagnosis, the villi has already recovered from not being exposed to gluten because you have already cut it out from your diet. This is completely counterproductive because now, you do not have an official diagnosis, your doctor may think that you are not being as honest in your discussions as he/she thought and your credibility is lost. Even though you may have Celiac Disease, the test results prove negative because you self diagnosed and self treated.

On the flip side, being armed with information can be very empowering. For example, when my daughter was going through her medical issues and very sick, I kept going in to various doctors and emergency rooms saying, "Something isn't right. I think it is more than just allergies. My mommy senses are tingling and I think we need to do some more tests." After saying this to one doctor in particular, he felt that I was "being dramatic and intentionally making my daughter sick to get attention" for myself. He admitted my daughter to the hospital for a 10 day "observation" period to prove to me that she was a healthy young girl with a couple allergies.

During that time I was not allowed to feed her anything that the hospital did not provide. They scheduled a round table meeting with us, her Pediatrician, Allergist, Gastroenterologist, and Child and Family Services. During this meeting I indicated that through my research I thought that she may possibly have Eosinophilic Esophagitis and asked them to perform a scope to see if she in fact did or did not. They chastised me and my husband for "looking for something" that really wasn't there and again accused me of intentionally making our daughter ill. I later found out that Child and Family Services was there to start the process to see if I was a fit mother or not.

A few days later, they performed the scope, and I will never forget the moment when the Gastroenterologist came out and said, "Your daughter has Eosinophilic Esophagitis". I remember where I was sitting, the sounds, and the smells. It still bothers me to walk by that spot when I go into that old hospital to visit someone else. But, I was right, they were wrong. Our Gastro-enterologist actually apologized to me for not listening to us and indicated that he learned a valuable lesson from us. The one doctor who admitted her for observation to prove that there was nothing wrong with her, dropped us from his case load (not that I complained). I never heard from Child and Family Services again.

The point of sharing this is to empower you and encourage you to do your research based on *creditable* information and speak with your doctor(s) armed with knowledge. But, don't jump the gun. If you look back at the symptoms listed in the above diseases/disorders, many of them overlap. You need your doctor's knowledge, skills, and diagnostic abilities to accurately diagnose you, just like we did with our daughter. We needed that scope done. I couldn't do it. My husband couldn't do it. Yet if I hadn't done my research and asked for it, who knows how much longer she would have suffered before we had a starting point in our journey.

CHAPTER TWO

Associated Health Issues

Nothing every runs perfectly. Not your car. Not your job. Not your body. Yes, things can run very smoothly for a long time, but everything has its bumps and glitches. Same is said for any food restrictive disease/disorder. Now that you have a bit of a handle on what your diagnosis means, it is time to start understanding some of the other issues that may go along with your disease/disorder.

Your body is one integrative system that is connected and intertwined in such a way that it only makes sense that when one organ or system is out of balance, or diseased, that other organs or systems may be affected. To what extent things are related is debated. Some people believe that you should treat each symptom individually. Other people take a more holistic approach and treat the person as a whole, seeing all the issues with your body and one combined issue that needs to be addressed. Yet others take a more spiritual approach by viewing the body as the final piece of your being that is affected and the problem is more deeply rooted.

Whatever your viewpoint, everyone can agree that there are some common health issues that go along with certain diseases/disorders. Taking a healthy approach to your lifestyle is very important in dealing with all of these diseases/disorders, and for your general health as well. Drinking enough water, getting enough exercise, managing stress levels, and especially watching your diet are all extremely important. By managing your lifestyle and taking a whole new approach to your health, you can live a full life. Taking this approach will never harm you or aggravate your symptoms, it will only improve them. Granted what is healthy for one person may not be the same as for another when you are dealing with chronic illness. It is highly individual and needs to be developed with your whole team.

Part of that healthy lifestyle is managing all of your symptoms and health issues to the best of your ability. If managing all of your symptoms means taking prescribed medication for a problem that has just arisen as a complication from your primary disease, or monitoring your seasonal allergies, then so be it.

Here is a partial discussion on some of the problems that may arise in conjunction with the previously discussed diseases/disorders. Again, this is not a complete list, just an overview of some of the more common ones that may pop up. This is meant to provide an overview for you, and as always, you can reference the last chapter for creditable resources to search on your own.

Asthma

DEFINITION: Asthma is chronic inflammation of the airway. In a normal lung, air is inhaled through the nose/mouth and passes through the trachea into large airways called bronchi.

From there the bronchi branch off into smaller tubes that have small sacs on the end called alveoli. The oxygen moves from the alveoli into the blood, while carbon dioxide is picked up from the blood. This is an easy process that should be automatic and not given much thought.

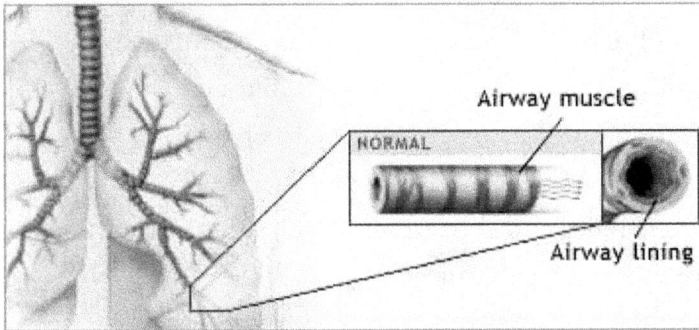

Normal

Airway muscle

NORMAL

Airway lining

(11)

In someone with asthma either the lining of the airways become inflamed and produces more mucous than usual, or the muscle that surrounds the airways tighten and twitch, causing the airways to narrow. Either way, the more inflamed the airways, the harder it is to pass air in and out of the lungs, making it difficult to breathe.

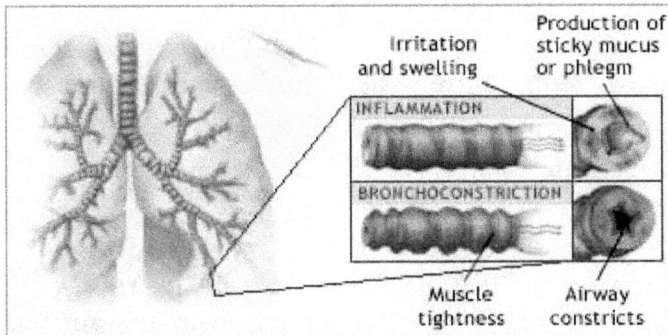

Asthmatic

Irritation
and swelling

Production of
sticky mucus
or phlegm

INFLAMMATION

BRONCHOCONSTRICTION

Muscle
tightness

Airway
constricts

(11)

SYMPTOMS: Symptoms arise when someone comes in contact with a "trigger". Triggers fall into two categories: Inflammatory (causing inflammation) and Symptom (non-allergic that generally do not cause inflammation but cause the airways to "twitch", made even worse if they are already inflamed).

Inflammatory Triggers	Symptom Triggers
• Air pollutants	• Air pollutants
• Moulds	• Cold air
• Pollens	• Exercise
• Viruses	• Smoke
• Cockroaches and dust mites	• Chemicals (perfumes, chemical smells, etc)
• Animals, especially fur bearing	• Strong emotions

For a person who has asthma, the symptoms vary in severity. Generally if you have a chronic cough, shortness of breath, wheezing, and/or a tight feeling in your chest, you are experiencing asthma symptoms. These symptoms may come and go. They may come on suddenly or gradually increase in intensity. This is when it is important to come up with an action plan with your doctor so that you are fully aware of what to do and when.

TREATMENT: As mentioned, treatment is highly individualized. You need to work closely with your doctor to determine what your triggers are, and avoid them, figure out what medication is required along with the proper dosage, and carry your reliever medication in case of an emergency. Medication for asthma falls into one of two categories.

The first is your controller medication, or preventer. This type of medication reduces the inflammation in the airways and is taken every day. You know your medication is working when one day you realize that you haven't had any symptoms for a while. The problem is, quite often people think, "Oh, I am symptom free! I don't need this anymore!" Wrong. Once you stop taking the medication, the inflammation may return. This is the point when you should see your doctor and maybe your dosage could be reduced or another option may be available, but do not stop taking your controller medication.

The second medication that you will be prescribed is your reliever medication. This type of medication helps control symptoms immediately if you are coughing or wheezing. They are short term solutions and do not solve the underlying problem of inflammation. If you are using your reliever medication increasingly, it is time to see your doctor because that is an indication that your asthma is getting worse and your controller medication may need to be changed.

ASSOCIATION: Asthma is most commonly associated with the following diseases/disorders:

- Allergies
- Eosinophilic Disorders

Constipation

DEFINITION: Most of us have probably suffered from this at one time or another, but no one really likes to talk about it. Constipation is the opposite of diarrhea; it is when your bowel movements become infrequent or difficult. Technically you are considered to be constipated if you have difficulty passing a stool at least a quarter of the time, have hard stools (refer to the Bristol Stool Chart in the appendix to see a comparison of what is considered hard, soft, etc.), or have less than three bowel movements in a week.

What is normal for one person may not be normal for another. You may have a bowel movement once a day, once every second day, or three times a day. But, if things start getting "un-normal", then you need to consider that you may be constipated.

So why would you become constipated in the first place? Some of the reasons for constipation are:

- Medications or supplements
- Not enough water daily
- Inadequate exercise
- Diet
- Stress
- Hemorrhoids (causing you to resist the urge to have a bowel movement due to the pain associated with them)

- Long term laxative use (weakens the muscles)
- Pregnancy
- Not going to the bathroom when the urge hits (common cause in children)

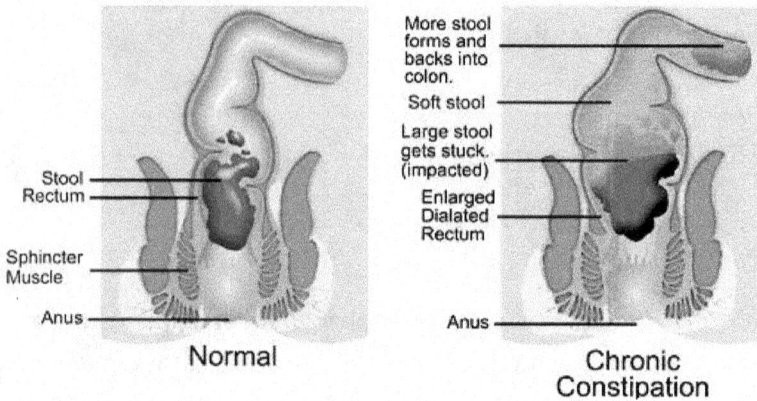

Normal

Chronic Constipation

(12)

SYMPTOMS: If you have ever been badly constipated, you know how bad the pain can be. In addition to pain, your tummy area can be swollen and/or tender and you can even feel nauseous or vomit from it. If you feel a persons' abdomen when they are constipated, you can even feel lumps in the large descending colon (you need to have them lay down and push relatively hard into the abdominal cavity).

TREATMENT: When you are constipated, you need to draw water into your colon to soften up the stools. You can do this very easily by drinking more water. Another thing that really helps things to get moving in your bowels is to move your whole body. Simple walking will help your muscles inside your body to move and get things flowing. So will eating a diet with plenty of natural fibre in it; fruits, vegetables, whole grains, cereals, prunes, and if necessary a fibre supplement such as psyllium husks or a product that has fibre in it (there are plenty on the market). Finally, if this doesn't work, then you can take a form of laxative that will draw water into your bowel and start things moving. Do not use a laxative for more than two weeks though because overuse can cause its own set of problems.

ASSOCIATION: Constipation is commonly found in Eosinophilic Disorders, Crohn's, Colitis, Food Intolerance, Food Allergies, and IBS. Although, most people will experience constipation at some point; the trick is to realize if it is associated with your particular disorder, or if it is just a normal course of life.

Dehydration

DEFINITION: We all know that we need to drink enough fluids every day. We also know that we lose fluids all the time due to regular bodily functions like sweating, breathing, etc. But, when we lose too much water, we become dehydrated and our bodies become out of balance. There can be various causes of dehydration, and without going into too much detail, they can be:

- Fever
- Not being able to drink
- Vomiting
- Diarrhea
- Increased urination
- Injuries to the skin such as burns, sores, oozing eczema, infection, etc
- Heat exposure
- Too much exercise

SYMPTOMS: As with anything, symptoms vary tremendously from minor to severe. Your scale of severity goes from an increase in thirst to death. Here is a breakdown of the different symptoms of dehydration:

- Urine color is deep yellow or orange rather than a pale yellow
- Dry mouth
- Dry skin
- Confusion
- Fainting
- Decreased urine output
- Inability to produce tears
- Dizziness
- Weakness
- Headache
- Confusion
- Inability to sweat
- Swollen tongue

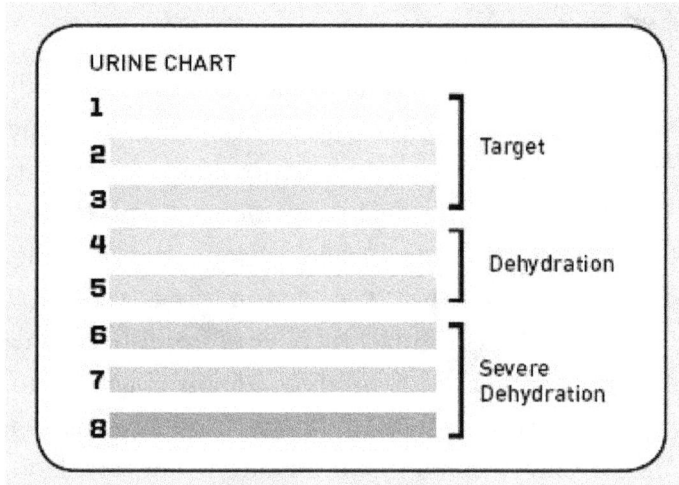

(13)

TREATMENT: You can treat mild to moderate dehydration at home by using one or more of these methods:

- Sipping small amounts of water
- Sucking on an ice cube/chips
- Sucking on popsicles made from fruit juice/sports drinks
- Drinking electrolyte containing drinks (homemade or store bought)

If the person has become dehydrated enough to warrant going to the emergency room, then they will generally give you an IV to replace fluids or supervised oral fluid replacement with electrolyte drinks.

ASSOCIATION: Dehydration can be associated with any of the diseases/disorders discussed in this book. It can also be associated with numerous conditions discussed in this chapter, in particularly diarrhea and eczema.

Diarrhea

DEFINITION: When we think of diarrhea, we generally think of the consistency of stools, rather than the frequency. But both are important to consider when talking about diarrhea. If you normally have two bowel movements a day, then sudden-ly start having four a day, then you would technically be considered to have diarrhea. Or, if your stools are much looser and/or waterier than normal, then you are also considered to have diarrhea. Most often these two categories are combined in people with diarrhea. Most of us can probably relate to that. Not only do you have to go more often, but you have much looser than normal stools.

The looseness of stools can be attributed to an increase in water in the stools. Normally, the lower portion of the small intes-tine, and the colon, absorb water from any undigested food that reaches that point. This creates a more or less solid stool with a definite form that passes easily through your final section of the gastrointestinal tract. If not enough water is absorbed as it goes through the process, if the stomach/small intestine secrete too much liquid, or if the undigested food passes too quickly through the gastrointestinal tract, then diarrhea results.

Diarrhea is divided into either acute (lasting 3 − 7 days) or chronic (lasts more than 3 weeks generally). It can be broken down into five types:

- Secretory Diarrhea − too much liquid is secreted into the intestine by the stomach or small intestine.
- Collagenous Colitis - the colon is unable to absorb fluid due to extensive scarring and/or inflammation.

- Motility Related Diarrhea – our intestines work by having small muscles contract along it moving the digested food through it. If these muscles are over active, then food is passed through too quickly not allowing enough time for the colon to absorb fluid as it passes through.

- Osmotic Diarrhea – small molecules pass into the intestine which draws water and electrolytes into the intestine.

- Inflammatory Diarrhea – the inflammation that causes this type of diarrhea can be caused from viruses, bacteria, toxins (such as food poisoning), or from diseases/disorders which cause inflammation of that organ, such as Colitis, Eosinophilic disorders, etc.

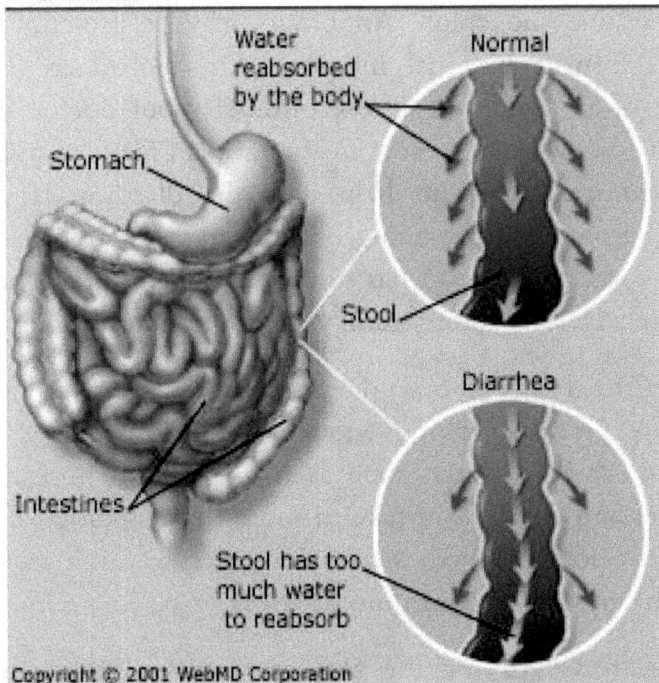

Diarrhea

Water reabsorbed by the body

Normal

Stomach

Stool

Diarrhea

Intestines

Stool has too much water to reabsorb

Copyright © 2001 WebMD Corporation

(14)

SYMPTOMS: The symptoms of diarrhea depend on the type and the severity of it. Symptoms can last from a few hours, to months depending on the cause. Here is a list of some of the symptoms that may arise from diarrhea:

- Pain
- Cramping
- Sense of urgency
- Fever
- Intestinal bleeding
- Dehydration

TREATMENT: Depending on the cause of the diarrhea, there are various treatment options for you. The first is over-the-counter medication to help stop the diarrhea. These work in one of two ways. The first is to slow down the muscle contraction of the intestine so that digested food does not move as quickly through it. The second form works by absorbing the excess water in the small intestine and colon. Antibiotics may be prescribed if the cause is from a bacterial infection. Or, if you are suffering because of an associated disease/disorder, your doctor and you may have to work on a new treatment plan for you and/or use prescribed medication to help with the diarrhea. If you are suffering from food poisoning or an allergic reaction to a food, then as soon as the food has stopped being ingested and it has completely cleared your system, you should return to normal.

Some of the things you can do at home to help with diarrhea is to ensure you are getting enough soluble fibre (the type of fibre that absorbs water, such as rice, psyllium husks, etc) in your diet and ensure you take in more than usual fluids. If it is a very bad bout of diarrhea, you may need to drink an electrolyte drink to restore your fluid balance.

ASSOCIATION: Any of the food restrictive diseases/disorders that have been covered in the first chapter can have diarrhea associated with it.

Eczema

DEFINITION: Eczema is a condition that is inflammatory in nature, chronic and is variable in the symptoms that are shown. It can occur anywhere on the skin, but most often it is seen in the areas of the body that have creases, such as the bends of arms, behind the knees, etc. There are different types of eczema, all of which can be triggered by stress.

- Atopic Eczema – this is the most common type and is associated with allergies and asthma. It occurs in both adults and children. In my experience, once the offending allergen has been removed, it will begin to clear up.

- Allergic Contact Dermatitis – this is caused by having an allergen contact your skin and generally happens over time. This is an immune system reaction similar to clinical allergies.

- Irritant Contact Dermatitis – this is caused from frequent contact with a chemical or detergent.

- Discoid Eczema – this is found in adults and are small round shaped patches of dry skin found on the lower body.

- Varicose Eczema – this is caused by poor circulation generally around the lower extremities of adults.

- Infantile Seborrheic Eczema – this is commonly known as cradle cap in infants under one year of age. It looks worse than it is. It generally isn't sore and itchy and does not seem to cause the baby any discomfort.

- Adult Seborrheic Eczema – this generally resembles dandruff in adults but can spread to surrounding areas of the head. It is thought to be caused by yeast growth and can become infected.

SYMPTOMS: Symptoms again vary in severity. Most often you will see dry patches that may ooze (if severe enough the oozing can cause dehydration), itch, be scaly, and are often red and inflamed. The eczema may "travel" meaning that as soon as one area clears up, it will appear in another area. Infection can occur at the site of eczema as well due to scratching, leaving the area open to bacteria.

TREATMENT: Treatment for eczema may include: medicated creams; moisturizing with creams, not lotions (lotions are primarily made of water, which evaporates, which in the long term actually dries out the area more); antifungal creams; and avoidance of any irritants/allergens. In my own personal experience, I find that drinking large amounts of water helps as well as a probiotic (friendly bacteria).

Eczema Prevention Tips

- Avoidance of over-bathing
- Applying moisturizer frequently, especially after bathing
- Bathing in warm, not hot, water and using a mild soap
- Limiting or avoiding contact with known irritants like soaps, perfumes, detergents, jewelry, environmental irritants, etc.
- Wearing loose-fitting clothing (cotton clothing may be less irritating for many people than wool or synthetic fibers)
- The use of cool compresses to help control itching
- Avoiding foods that cause allergic reactions

(15)

ASSOCIATION: Eczema is most often associated with Food Allergies, Eosinophilic Disorders, and sometimes Food Intolerances.

Edema

DEFINITION: Edema is a fancy way of saying swelling. This is caused by an excess amount of fluid trapped in the tissues of your body. This is quite often found in ankles, hands, feet, and legs. The reason fluid builds up in your tissues is from different medications, pregnancy, or a disease that you may have.

SYMPTOMS: If you have edema, then you will notice that there is swelling or puffiness directly under your skin which can appear stretched or shiny. You may notice that your abdomen has increased in size as a result of your organs taking on excess fluid as well. A good test to see if you have edema is to press on the affected area with your finger for a few seconds and then let go. If a dimple, or indent, remains then you have edema.

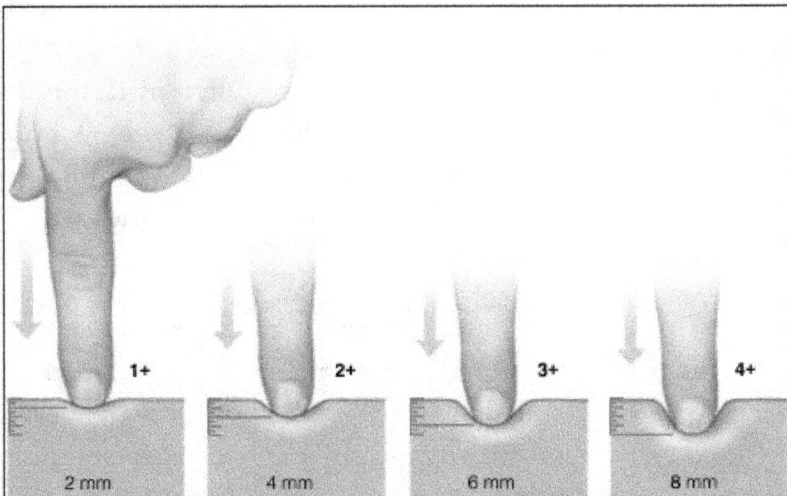

(16)

TREATMENT: One of the easiest treatments for edema is to watch your salt intake. The salt will draw fluid into your tissues and hold it there. If you have less salt in your diet (generally less than 2000 mg per day) then this should help. You may also need to take medication to help remove the excess fluid if it is bad enough.

ASSOCIATION: Edema can be associated with any of the diseases/disorders mentioned in the previous chapter, from any medication you may be taking associated with it or from your body being out of balance. It is also associated most commonly with Diabetes, Food Allergies, and Eosinophilic Disorders.

Rash/Hives

DEFINITION: A rash is a general term to describe an outbreak on the skin that is inflamed, itchy and usually red. They are caused by allergic reactions, medication side effect, infections, or sometimes for unknown reasons. A hive is a swollen red bump on the skin that appears suddenly and can be limited to one, or appear in clumps. Hives are a result of histamine being released by the body caused from many different factors such as allergic reactions, chemicals, medication, extreme hot or cold, or sunlight exposure. You may not always know what caused the rash or hive, and there may not always be an explanation for it.

SYMPTOMS: Generally speaking, rashes and hives are very itchy – sometimes to the point of scratching so much you break the skin. If you have ever had these, you know how unbearable they can be! Other than the itch you can also get muscle soreness, edema, redness and localized swelling. If you have any breathing problems, tightness in your chest, or difficulty speaking/swallowing, then the symptoms are indicative of a much more serious allergic reaction and immediate medical attention needs to be sought out.

TREATMENT: Depending on the severity of the rash/hive you can try a few different tricks. First of all, antihistamines work great and should be used for the more severe reactions. Cool cloths placed on the rash help with the itch as well, so does apple cider vinegar (place a few drops on a cotton ball and apply to affected area). Aloe Vera gel not only relieves sunburns but it works well for treating a rash, as long as you aren't allergic to it. Having a bath in an oatmeal can help with any itch, again, as long as you aren't allergic to it.

There are many over-the-counter remedies for itches and rashes, as well as numerous home remedies. The trick is to find one that works for you and is most comfortable. I remember bathing my daughter in oatmeal baths and putting oatmeal lotions on her as a baby to try and help with the itch and it never seemed to help. Then I realized she was allergic to it!

ASSOCIATION: Rashes and hives are generally associated with your food allergies, Eosinophilic Gastrointestinal Disorders, PKU and periodically food intolerances.

Reflux

DEFINITION: Reflux is a term used to describe what happens when the acid in your stomach moves up into your esophagus due to the sphincter (or ring of muscles) between the lower part of your esophagus and stomach not closing properly. If it is chronic, then it is referred to Gastroesophageal Reflux Disease (GERD).

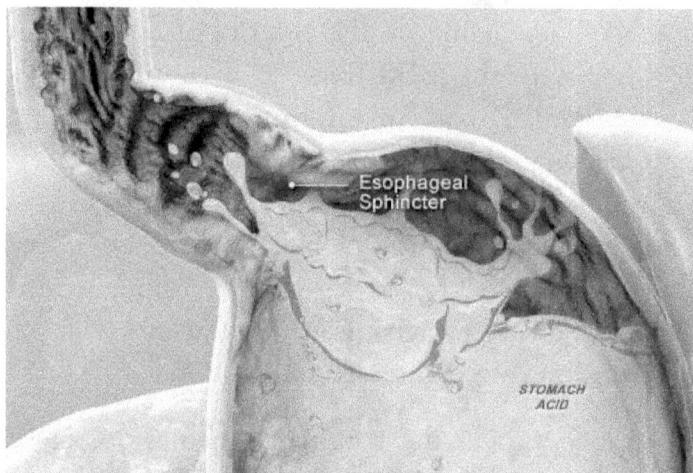

(35)

SYMPTOMS: The most common symptoms of reflux are heartburn (or pain that moves from your stomach to your chest area) and regurgitation (a horrible tasting acid that comes up into the back of your throat or mouth). Less common symptoms of reflux are burping, bloating, feeling like food is stuck in your throat, hiccups, nausea, and/or chronic sore throat.

TREATMENT: There are some changes to your diet and lifestyle that you can make that can help alleviate symptoms such as avoiding foods that are known to cause problems, eating smaller meals, raise the head of your bed by 5 inches or so, wear non-restrictive clothing, exercise, and if overweight, lose the weight. There are over the counter remedies as well, or if necessary your doctor may prescribe medication to help with the symptoms.

(34)

ASSOCIATION: Reflux is associated with Eosinophilic Gastro-intestinal Disorders, Diabetes, Allergies/Intolerances, Celiac Disease, IBS, and PKU. Keep in mind though that anyone can have a bought of reflux and it *not* be related to the disease/disorder that they are diagnosed with; just like anyone can get a sore throat, regardless if you have Eosinophilic Esophagitis or not.

Vitamin/Mineral Deficiency

DEFINITION: Vitamin/mineral deficiency is cause by one of two ways; either you are not taking in enough vitamins/minerals or your body is not able to absorb the vitamins/minerals properly. If the levels of vitamins/minerals are low enough, long enough, then problems can occur. Your body is an amazing machine though... it will do everything in its power not to let you become deficient in a certain vitamin or mineral by taking it from whatever source it can to keep you healthy. That is why it generally takes a while for symptoms to show.

Many of the foods we can purchase today are fortified or enriched with basic vitamins to ensure that most of the general population does not suffer from deficiencies, yet many of you who need to restrict your foods are not getting these vitamins/minerals from typical sources, so you need to pay particular attention to this and take proper steps to make sure you are getting all the nutrition you require.

SYMPTOMS: The symptoms of vitamin/mineral deficiency vary incredibly and can cause minor symptoms like a fishy body odor, or a major symptom like liver damage. The first chart is a condensed list of the major vitamins, the deficiency that can be caused, and good food sources of that vitamin. The first ten are water soluble vitamins (meaning they dissolve in water) and the last four are fat soluble vitamins (meaning they need to be consumed with other fats to be metabolized). The second chart goes over some of the major minerals in our diet.

Vitamin	Deficiency	Food Sources
Thiamin	Beriberi (condition that causes weight loss, weakness, pain in limbs, edema, irregular heartbeat, impaired sensory perception, and gastrointestinal problems amoung other issues)	Pork, whole grains, legumes, fortified/ enriched foods, tuna, and soy milk
Riboflavin (B2)	Ariboflavinosis (sore throat, cracked lips, dermatitis, decreased red blood cell count, and swollen mouth are most common)	Liver, mushrooms, dairy products, fortified/enriched foods, tomatoes and spinach
Niacin (B3)	Pellagra (skin lesions, weakness, mental confusion, aggression, diarrhea, dermatitis, insomnia are some symptoms)	Liver, fish, meat, fortified/enriched foods, tomatoes, and mushrooms
Pantothenic acid (B5)	Burning feet syndrome (severe burning and aching of the feet, generally on the bottom)	Liver, mushrooms, sunflower seeds, fortified foods, yogurt and turkey
Vitamin B6	Microcytic hypochromic anemia (red blood cells are smaller than normal and filled with less hemoglobin than usual)	Fish, chickepeas, liver, fortified foods, potatoes, and bananas
Biotin	Depression, loss of muscle control, and skin irritation	Peanuts, almonds, mushrooms, egg yolks, tomatoes, and avocados
Folate	Macrocytic anemia (blood cells are larger than normal)	Organ meats, legumes, okra, leafy vegetables, and fortified/enriched foods

Vitamin	Deficiency	Food Sources
Vitamin B12	Macrocytic anemia (blood cells are smaller than normal)	Mollusks, liver, salmon, meat, fortified foods, and cottage cheese
Vitamin C	Scurvy (weakness, lethargy, shortness of breath, bone pain, skin changes, gum disease, and poor wound healing)	Peppers, papayas, citrus fruit, broccoli, strawberries, and brussel sprouts
Choline	Liver damage	Eggs, liver, legumes, and pork
Vitamin A	Night blindness, failure to produce tears, and thickening of the skin	Liver, pumpkin, sweet potato and carrot
Vitamin D	Rickets (dental problems, muscle weakness, bone tenderness/fractures, deformity, low calcium levels in blood, soft skull, and widening of the wrist are typical symptoms); Osteomalacia (softening of the bones); and Osteoporosis (low bone mass and/or deterioration of bone)	Fish, shitake mushrooms, fortified milk and fortified cereals
Vitamin E	Neuromuscular problems (nerve impulses don't relay the information properly to your muscles causing a variety of symptoms depending on nerves affected); Hemolytic anemia (red blood cells are destroyed prematurely causing fatigue, pain and irregular heartbeats)	Tomatoes, nuts, seeds, spinach, and fortified cereals
Vitamin K	Causes problems with the blood clotting properly	Kale, spinach, broccoli, and brussel sprouts

(36)

Mineral	Deficiency	Food Sources
Calcium	Rickets (see description above); osteopenia (loss of bone mass); osteoporosis ; muscle pain/spasms; and tingling in hands/feet	Dairy products, dark green leafy vegetables, salmon, sardines (with bones), legumes, and fortified foods.
Phosphorus	Loss of appetite, anemia, muscle weakness and poor bone development	Dairy products, meat, seafood, nuts, and seeds
Magnesium	Abnormal nerve and muscle function, especially of the heart	Green leafy vegetables, seafood, legumes, nuts, dairy products, chocolate and whole grains
Sodium and Chloride	Electrolyte loss from diarrhea and/or vomiting causing nausea, dizziness, muscle cramps, and fatigue	Table salt, processed foods, meats, seafood, dairy products, poultry, condiments
Potassium	Can result from diarrhea and vomiting causing muscle weakness, constipation, irritability and confusion.	Legumes, potatoes, seafood, dairy products, meat, fruits and vegetables

(36)

TREATMENT: The severity of the deficiency dictates the treatment. I personally believe that preventing deficiencies is the best way to go to begin with, which is why I feel so strongly about people who need to restrict their foods working with a certified/registered/licensed nutritionist or dietician. As you can see from the above charts, some of the problems associated with vitamin/mineral deficiencies can be quite severe. At the very least, taking a high quality multivitamin can help you if you are required to restrict your foods, especially if there are multiple foods being restricted.

You will notice that I have not addressed deficiencies in protein, carbohydrates, or lipids (fats). This was not an over-sight. If I addressed these issues, then this 'short, sweet, to the point book" would be a university text book. Deficiencies in any of these macro nutrients can be catastrophic and need to be addressed on an individual basis, especially patients with PKU or Eosinophilic Disorders. Depending on the case, specialized formulas will be prescribed to help ensure that these key nutrients are being provided.

ASSOCIATION: Deficiencies can be associated with all of the diseases/disorders I have discussed in this book.

CHAPTER THREE

You and Your Medical Team

I am honestly blessed. I have a team surrounding my children that is amazing. Without them, I don't think that I would be as confident in myself when it comes to caring for my children. I have the type of relationship with them where they respect my opinion, knowledge, and experience; and I respect theirs. They work together, even though they are in different hospitals/offices, and the lines of communication are open all across the board. I didn't always have this amazing team, if you recall my earlier recollection of learning of my daughters' diagnosis, but I do now and I want to let them all know how much I appreciate them.

My wish for you is to get a team surrounding you and/or your loved one that will work with you and keep the lines of communication open. It will make your journey so much easier and less stressful. But please remember, we are all human. We all have good days and bad days. We all make mistakes, even professionals. Just as you want them to be patient and understanding with you – you need to return the courtesy.

So how do you go about building this amazing team and then work with them? I'll admit it may not always be easy. But if you try a few of these tips, you may find it easier than just hoping you get a great team.

Do Your Research and Ask for Referrals

Your family doctor is a general practice physician who will make referrals to specialists like Gastroenterologists, Allergists, Neurologists, etc as he/she feels fit. If you suspect that your child may need a referral to a specialist, then look up doctors in your area that work in that particular field. There are many websites that provide doctor references for you to read over. Read the comments and that can give you a general feel for what type of doctor he/she is. You may not always have the opportunity to ask your family doctor for a particular specialist, but you can ask questions, such as, "does that specialist work specifically with children?" If not, ask your family doctor if she/he does know of one and say that you heard that "Dr. So-And-So" does, is "Dr. So-And-So" accepting new patients?

Sometimes, a referral needs to be made to a hospital or clinic in general. If that is the case, you may not always have a choice of specialist, but you may have a choice of hospital. If that is the case, you may be able to request a certain hospital based on your research. For example, for Eosinophilic Disorders, there are a few hospitals in the USA that have a well established team that has extensive experience working with the disorder. If you had to be referred for a scope to look for that disorder in particular, you may be able to request a referral to one of those centers over another one that is not as well versed in Eosinophilic Disorders.

Different countries, states, or provinces have different protocols for referrals and looking for doctors. If you are able to "shop around" for a doctor, you may want/need to. Not everyone has that option, so you'll have to do the best you can. And don't be afraid to ask the doctor you are seeing, knowing that he/she is not a good fit for you, if they could refer you to another doctor who may be able to help you.

When we moved to a different city, I asked my current Gastroenterologist (whom I just gained a huge amount of respect for and vice versa) to refer me to the best Gastroenterologist he knew of in the new city we were moving to – and he didn't fail me. From there, he introduced me to other professionals to work with and build a relationship with. Now, I am lucky enough to say that I consider some of these people my friends, and we look forward to our appointments so that we can catch up.

Be Humble and Honest

You have done your research on the disease/disorder that is affecting you or your loved one. You have the tools to make better decisions than you did before. But remember, nobody knows everything and you can always learn more. If you go into your appointments thinking and acting like you know it all, the response you get will not be as respectful as if you approach each appointment as a chance to have a dialog and learn from each other. Think of the last time you had a conversation with a "know-it-all". How did you feel? How did you react? How could it have gone better? Those thoughts, feelings and reactions are exactly what your doctor will be going through if you go into the appointment on an arrogant note.

Part of being humble is knowing that you have more to learn, so ask questions that are relevant and intelligent. If you don't understand what was just said, then ask for clarification. If there is a procedure that is going to happen, and you have never seen the inside of an Operating Room before and you are feeling nervous, ask if you can have a tour before the procedure to ease your nerves if that is what it takes.

Please don't be afraid to ask questions. The worst that can happen is someone will say no. You are no further behind than you were before you asked.

Be prepared

Before you appointment, it will always make things easier and smoother if you come fully prepared. If you are just starting your journey in searching for a diagnosis, make sure you have a list of your symptoms, when they happen, etc. There are forms in the Appendix that may help you track this. There is nothing worse than having your time wasted, same goes for a doctor. If you go in saying, "I just don't feel good and I want to know what's wrong", then the doctor doesn't have much to go on. But, if you have a clear list of symptoms, patterns, and as much detail as possible, especially when you are dealing with gastro-intestinal issues, then your doctor will be better informed to help you out. Also, having a list will help you remember everything. It is so easy to forget one or two things when you are having a conversation with a doctor because other topics will come up and the dialog will take on a life of its' own. I can't count how many times I have left a doctor's office and thought, "shoot! I forgot to tell him about ....." Please learn from my mistake and save yourself some grief.

Show Respect

This should go without saying. Doctors and specialists are very well educated, and have years of experience under their belt. That counts for a lot. But, they are also human and all humans have a limited amount of knowledge that they can store in that magnificent brain. Even though you may be frustrated that you don't get an immediate answer to your health question/problem, you need to understand that there are tests to be done and sometimes even research to be done.

Sometimes, in order to make a diagnosis, other diseases/disorders need to be ruled out. Periodically that means that a treatment will be started to see if it works. If not, then that is not the problem. A perfect example is Eosinophilic Esophagitis. In order to make this diagnosis, one of the criteria is to treat the person for reflux and not respond to it. Frustrating course of action, but necessary. For you parents out there, how many times have you said to your child(ren), "don't ask why, I have my reasons". Same goes for the doctor treating you. Even though you may be certain that you have Eosinophilic Esophagitis, he/she needs to rule out reflux first.

Again, we are all human. People like certain types of people, while they dislike others. Just because you may or may not "like" your doctor, or any other part of your medical team, that doesn't mean that you should not respect them. You are not expected to always like everybody. Shoot! You can't tell me that you always like every member of your own family all the time. But, it will help your relationship with your doctor/specialist/dietician/nutritionist/etc, if you show them the respect that they rightly deserve. And they will most likely in turn, show you the same respect.

Don't Be Scared

When talking with my kids (currently 6 and 11) about this chapter, I asked them if they could offer any piece of advice to people about working with their medical team, what would it be? Their response was simple, "Don't be scared, they are just trying to help you." How simple; how true. This is especially true of any procedures that you may have to go through. My daughter has gone through more testing/procedures than my husband and I combined, from the age of 4 months. Not once did she cringe in fear. I did as her mother, but she has always been a brave little soul. My son is the same. A big part of it I think, is how my husband and I reacted. If we showed our fear in front of them, I am sure that they would have fed off of it and been scared. But we always waited until we were out of ear/eye shot to show our own fears and anxiety.

Yes, there will be scary times, like heading into an operating room, holding your child as he/she is put under anesthesia and going limp in your arms, or even getting that first stitch in a cut eye. But how you deal with it will determine how the experience will go.

Think about it, would your child like to see her parents bawling and freaking out while she gets a scope done, or would she rather see smiling faces with warm loving eyes looking at her as she gets wheeled off to the procedure room? What would you rather see? Rest assure that the people caring for your child are absolutely amazing. That is why they work in a children's hospital. They have been around the block. They know how to make a child feel at ease. And if it is you, same applies.

I remember when I had my son, and the epidural didn't take, I had a choice. Make jokes and laugh about the whole situation, or focus on the pain. It was a lot more fun because I made jokes and bugged them about wanting pizza and beer as soon as it was over. Don't get me wrong, it hurt like the dickens, but at least I have fond memories of that day rather than needing to apologize to my husband for the cruel things I said/did. Or the day, my dad went in for his 12 hour surgery to put in his artificial heart. There was a huge chance we would never see him again. As a family, we made the choice to leave him with hugs, smiles and a, "see you in a few hours". Thankfully we did.

Medical Procedures

I touched on this previously, but there are some tips/tricks to help you get through them, whether it is yourself, or your child. When it comes to having a procedure or operation done, your doctor, and your surgeon, will explain what will happen. This is your chance to ask as many questions as you want or need to. If you are like me, you want to know everything. Or, if you prefer to just know the basics, then that is fine. I firmly believe though that knowledge is power. If you know exactly what is going to happen, how long it is going to take, etc., then there is nothing to be nervous about. This goes back to when I was a young child and my dad started having his heart troubles. I would ask questions and get as much information as I could so that I knew what could happen and why. That way if it did, then I was already prepared to handle it. Similar to taking first aid, you hope you never need to use it, yet if you do need it, it is readily available in your memory bank.

When children are involved, the people at children's hospitals are amazing. They know how to explain what is going on in language your child can understand, without scaring them.

Sometimes, they will pull out the old teddy bear and show them what happens on the teddy bear. They have even been known to give a tour of the procedure/operating room if asked. If you would like more information, or a tour, or anything, just ask. The worst that can happen is they will say no. But remember to show that respect when having these types of conversations.

And a bonus that a lot of people sometimes forget about... after a procedure, especially an esophageal scope, you get a popsicle!

Be Your Own Advocate

Because honestly, who else is going to be? Or who will advocate for your child if you don't? Being an advocate doesn't mean holding sit-ins or tying yourself to someone's desk. It means speaking up for yourself and pleading your own case, especially if there are extenuating circumstances that require financial assistance through different agencies. This can be a tough one. Sometimes you will have to be "pleasantly persistent" as I have once been referred to.

There is a fine line here that cannot be crossed, especially when dealing with a team of professionals that you will potentially be working with for years. But if you are well informed, courteous, and honest, then advocating for yourself or your loved one is easy, if even necessary at all.

Remember Your Pharmacist

Quite often people overlook this very important person in their life, and that is a shame. When it comes to pharmacological agents, this is the expert. When it comes to non-medicinal ingredients, this is the expert, especially if you have food allergies. When it comes to knowing all of the side effects of a drug, the duration of the drug, and whether or not to take it with food, this is the expert.

Your pharmacist has the ability to contact your physician to get the prescription changed if there is an ingredient in it that you can't have. For example, my daughter's physician prescribed a tablet form of a drug that she needed. I dutifully asked the pharmacist to check for non-medicinal ingredients because it was new and sure enough lactose was the first ingredient. He then called the doctor to request that he could substitute the liquid form that did not have the lactose in it. Because of my relationship that I built with our local pharmacist, it was an easy exchange and we prevented an anaphylactic reaction. I hate to think what the outcome could have been if it weren't for this integral person in our team.

Thank Goodness for Nurses

These men and women are the front line workers, and unfortunately we all have a stereotypical image in our head of nurses with all the time in the world to just tend to you. Not so much. These amazing people have a lot of patients to look after, enormous amounts of paperwork, and get stuck with all the dirty jobs. I have always made an effort to show my appreciation each and every time I am working with a nurse, especially in a hospital setting. If you can help out in any way possible do it. If there is no reason that you can't go to the patient fridge to get your own juice – then do it. For all you know your nurse is also looking after another patient who is currently violently vomiting. And with all due respect, that is a little more important at this instant than you being lazy and not getting your own juice.

One friend of mine who is a nurse at a major hospital in Edmonton let me in on a few behind the scene goings-on in the day of a nurse, one of them being just coming off a 24 hour shift because they were so short staffed. Keep that in mind next time you find yourself losing patience with the front line workers; there is a lot more going on that what is happening in your situation. And even though what you are going through is extremely important, it may not be as critical as what somebody else is going through at the exact same time that requires attention.

CHAPTER FOUR

Family, Friends, and Social Gatherings

I must say, I have been blessed with a very supportive, loving, caring and understanding family, both immediate and extended. Without them, I am sure this journey we have gone on, and continue, would not be as smooth as it has been and will be. That being said, I have talked with many people who aren't so blessed. From talking with these people, and learning from my own experiences, hopefully this chapter will help you pave the road to a lifelong journey, because that is what it is. Chronic food restrictions are a lifelong thing. It will change a little over time, or even drastically. Symptoms will come and they will go. Having your family, immediate and extended, as well as close friends, be a part of your journey will make everyone's life that much less complicated.

Family

Family is such an open term now because of the society we live in and I love that! If you noticed in my dedication, I have three parents and I am fortunate enough to be able to include all of them in each and every function we have. As a child growing up, I was always able to call on whichever one I needed most at the time (or whichever one I thought would give me what I wanted ...). Now that I have a family of my own, my definition of family has changed, because I have added my own children, a step mother and my in-laws to the mix. I didn't think it possible, but now I have six parents! And more sisters! And brothers-in-law! I love how even the simple stable things in life can change.

But for some families, their family may include mom, aunt and brother; or dad, dad and the family dog; or just you and your significant other; or you and your dearest friend; even just you and your child. Whatever wonderful combination you refer to as your family, that is who am talking about here. Their understanding, support, and patience is so important to your health, or the health of your loved one, that I really wanted to emphasize this.

Being able to go through this process on a daily basis with someone makes it a little more bearable. If you are a parent and going through doctor's appointments, tests, procedures, waiting, and maybe tears with your child, being able to share this with someone will help. It will also help in the long run as you all learn to live with this new life of reading labels, managing symptoms, future tests and appointments and anything else that you will have to prepare your child to someday manage on his/her own.

It also helps to learn new things with a partner because in the beginning there will be a huge amount of information you will have to digest, and having somebody else digest it with you will make it easier to remember down the road. That, and two brains are better than one when it comes to remembering and/or coming up with new ideas.

And one thing to remember is that if you are a parent with a child going through the process of finding out what is going on, remember that you are not the only one who loves your child and cares about him/her. Your family is just as concerned and worried as you are most likely. They may not say it or show it much (and that could very likely be from not wanting to create more stress/anxiety for you or bother you) but they do in their own way. So please remember to keep the lines of communication open with them. And honesty is the best policy. From personal experience, I have learned that being on the receiving end of "trying not to hurt or worry" someone, actually creates more problems because the person you are trying to protect is ultimately being lied to, and nobody appreciates that – regardless of the reason.

If you are the one who is being/has been diagnosed then all the same applies. The only difference really is that you don't have to watch another person going through all this and worry about, just yourself; doesn't always make it easier though.

Remember those lectures you used to get as a kid about, "put yourself in their shoes", or 'be nice, you don't know what they are going through", or "just because it doesn't seem like a big deal to you, it may be to them", repeat them to yourself often. Everyone deals with situations differently, especially if they are stressful or new to them. Even more so if it means giving up cheesecake for the rest of your life.

Here are some quick tips to help you and your family navigate:

- Make the focus of meal/celebration time on the people around you and the conversations that can be had – not on the food.
- Be patient with each other

- Remember that if you aren't submerged in it every day, it is easy to forget, especially if there are numerous food restrictions. My children have never been able to have an ice cream cone, yet my dad still suggests going to get ice cream on a nice day, then catches himself.

- Don't get mad at each other for what you may consider "common knowledge". For example if you have a milk allergy you are fully aware that "casein" is an ingredient to avoid on labels, whereas your brother who sees you once every four months is unaware.

- Be a patient teacher. Take them grocery shopping and teach them how to read labels. Show them how administer insulin or whatever medication may be required. Try and bring up memories of their worst tummy ache to give them something to reference for the pain you may be going through. Whatever method works best for whatever needs to be taught should be done, and done patiently with love. Sometimes this is easier said than done, especially if it is for the third, fourth, etc time, but do your best.

- Don't set them up for failure. If your sister wants to make dinner for you and you are celiac, don't leave it up to her to research ingredients etc. Offer to help, provide brand names of products that you know are safe, and offer some of your favourite recipes. Whatever you can do to make that dinner as safe and wonderful as possible should be done. You don't want to create a situation where you get sick, she feels guilty and incompetent, and the whole evening is ruined.

- You know what it is like to receive a guilt trip – don't give one. It does absolutely no good. If something arises that didn't go well, deal with it in a mature, up-front manner.

It may not be easy, but it is always best in the long run. There will be potential problems enough in the future, you don't want to create any unnecessarily.

- Show honest, genuine appreciation for their support and effort, no matter how small. We all like to hear "thank-you". The effort of accommodating food restrictions, especially when you are not used to it, is huge. Who knows, maybe Sunday dinner has always included Grandma's fresh baked buns for 50 years, but she didn't do it this time, just because you cannot eat them. A simple, "thanks Grandma for not making buns for dinner tonight on my behalf" goes a long way.

Friends

Thank goodness for friends! They are there for you to talk to, cry to, yell at, or whatever you need. They are there to provide you with a break if you need, and even give you a distraction from your own worries. Some will completely understand your health issues, some won't; but regardless they are an invaluable resource. And each friend will be a different resource. One friend you can call on to babysit if you need. Another will go out with you and make you laugh until you cry. Yet another you feel safe enough with to allow them to cook you or your loved ones dinner.

The best way to approach your food restrictions with friends, is similar to family – after all, many of us consider our friends to be as close as family anyhow. But, they aren't. So, when it comes to gruesome details of your latest procedure, I don't know if that is something you necessarily want to share. So, use your best judgement, and still be honest.

Social Gatherings

I'm not going to lie; these can be tough when you need to restrict your foods for whatever reason. Think about it, how many social occasions can you think of that don't involve food in some manner? Birthdays, holidays, weddings, informal gatherings, kindergarten graduation, high school graduation, the list can go on and on. The trick is be prepared, be creative, and prepare those around you.

For example, my children are severely restricted in the foods they can eat. For my daughter's first birthday, the only food she could tolerate was sweet potato. That was all she could eat. No seasonings, no icing, no nothing. So, I found a big sweet potato, cooked it up, cut it into a cylindrical shape, and "iced" it with mashed sweet potato. Then I "decorated" it with little homeopathic white tablets that we were trying. Or my son, for his first birthday he could only have rice. So, I made homemade marshmallow fluff, colored it with grey food coloring, and mixed it together with rice puffs. Then I filled a toy (new and washed) dump truck and front end loader with the "dirt". Not your typical birthday cake, but they still got to enjoy a first birthday, make a mess, get spoiled by grandparents, and be surrounded by those who love them most. Isn't that what a birthday is really supposed to be about anyway?

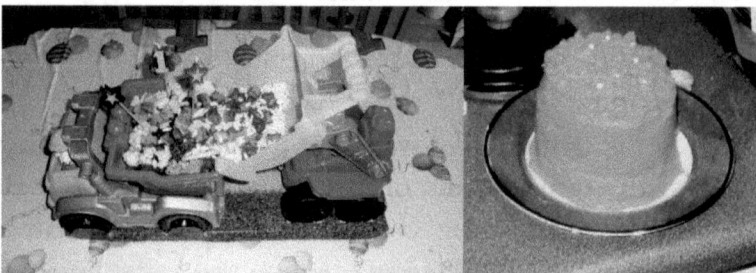

I was so proud of my husband this year, because when it comes to the cooking and creativity – that generally falls on my plate, even when it comes to me. I even have to make my own birthday cakes. But this year for my birthday, I was the one who couldn't eat much... so he made me a birthday "cake" that has never been better! A hollowed out honeydew melon, filled with strawberries, "iced" with coconut spread, and drizzled with Nestle® Nesquik. Even managed the candles! (For future reference, coconut spread is more like margarine and not an icing for those of you who are considering it...) First time in my life that I didn't feel guilty about eating my whole birthday cake, less the coconut spread!

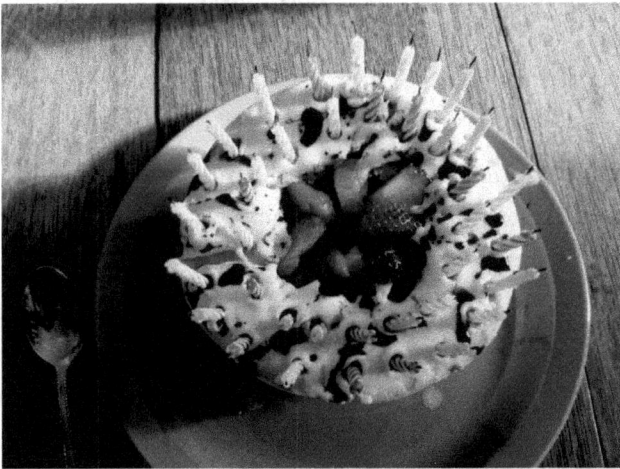

Celebrations are relatively easy for me, because I am in control of the ingredients, utensils, etc. and my extended family is very understanding and have no issue with me hosting most of the holidays and events. Yes, the work load can be insane. I have been known to cook three separate meals for one occasion. But that is a fair trade off for the reduced stress level going out causes for everyone involved. But what do you do when you are invited out to a celebration where there is food, or your child is invited to a birthday party with a bunch of kids running around with food? Here are some tips to make it a little less stressful:

- Talk with the host as soon as possible to find out what the menu is going to be like. If you discern that there is nothing safe, ask permission to bring your own food. If there are a few things that will be safe, still be wary.

- If it is a child's birthday party, often there will be decorations on the cake/cupcake. Ask if you may have one to decorate the dessert you will be bringing so that your child feels included.

- Again, with a child's birthday party, if they are giving out goody bags, request that one be made for your child without food items in it, and always check it before you allow your child to have anything in it.

- If the host offers to make something that is safe for you or your loved one, offer to help, or offer up some name brands of items you know are safe.

- If you are going to a restaurant, look at the menu in advance to see what items you have to choose from. Call ahead and let them know that you are coming and have food allergies/celiac/etc. Most places are very helpful and considerate when you indicate that you cannot have an ingredient.

- Bring your own food, just in case. I have a 12v cooler in the back of my truck that I always have stocked with safe foods, water and the formula my kids need. I even have plastic cutlery that I know is not contaminated in there. Granted, ¾ of us can't stop at the local Tim Hortons® to grab something, so it is imperative I am prepared.

You have probably noticed a common theme starting to weave its way into these pages... be prepared. When it comes to your health, is it really worth not eating the fresh bowl of berries covered in whipped cream for dessert or asking if the steak your friend grilled for you has been basted with butter if you are intolerant to dairy? Or even worse, not even asking because you are afraid to offend someone? Think about how that person may feel if you didn't ask and ended up having to be admitted to the hospital because of something they fed you.

CHAPTER FIVE

Emotions Surrounding Food Restrictions

As I mentioned previously, this isn't easy, especially if you have to restrict multiple ingredients. It is even harder, I think, if you have been able to eat a certain way for years, decades even, and then all of a sudden you need to omit a food group. I often say that my kids are lucky because they have never tasted a cheesecake and therefore they don't know what they are missing. When they see a commercial on TV for a burger covered in bacon and cheese with mushrooms spilling out the edge, their mouths don't salivate like mine does.

We are constantly inundated with food images and smells, and for someone who has dietary restrictions this can be a form of torture – if you let it. Walking through a mall, passing by the food court can be excruciating, unless you learn to take it for what it is – an aroma that smells pleasant. That's it. My husband thinks I'm crazy because I will ask to smell his chocolate muffin, just like I ask a florist if I can smell the roses in her shop. The food is an object that smells great. I know that if I were to eat it, I would be in agony. I learned that lesson the hard way. But, I have changed my perspective and I hope that you can get to that point.

Again, it isn't easy, especially if you are an adult. You have had years of eating foods and being socialized to associate food with good times. You need to learn, and teach those around you, that it isn't the food that creates the good times, it is the good times that creates good memories. When you get right down to it, food exists for one reason, to provide us nourishment. It isn't here to provide us with holidays, memories, and celebrations. It is here to fuel our body so that we can grow, flourish, and enjoy life. If you are a Celiac, are you going to grow, flourish and enjoy life if you eat that fresh baked bread that just came out of the oven? No. You will be lying on the couch in pain while life carries on without you.

In order to emotionally deal with food restrictions, you need to change your mind set. You need to deconstruct the most basic things you know and reconstruct them in a way that makes sense in your new world. A world that doesn't necessarily exist for everyone, but does exist for you and others out there who need to restrict their diets. Don't get me wrong, I have been brought to tears grocery shopping looking at all the wonderful snacks for kids that I can't buy for my own kids. The trick is, when times like this pop up, you need to accept that it happened, deal with it, and move on.

Once you/your loved one receive a diagnosis of (fill in the blank) you will inevitably go through a process. This process, I believe, is very similar to the five stages of grieving:

1   *Denial and Isolation* – you will go through an overwhelming rush of emotions all mixed together. You will feel defeated, angry, strong, weak, determined, confused,

overwhelmed, exhausted, elated, and the list goes on. One minute you may be crying, the next you are in autopilot, and then you are completely zoned out. You will also feel like you are the only one in the world who is going through this. But remember, you are not alone. There are others out there who are going through the same thing and can help you through this stage. Support groups are everywhere for many of the diseases/disorders that I talk about in this book in addition to others. This stage is usually fairly temporary, but can range from days to years, depending on each person. For me, with my daughter, it lasted about a year. With my son, it lasted about a day because I was already used to it. But when I was diagnosed, the denial lasted a few months. This just goes to show, that it is not a onetime occurrence, because nothing ever happens in a vacuum.

2 *Anger* – why me? Why do I have to go through this? Why can't they find a cure or a pill to fix this? Why don't more restaurants provide more options? Why don't my friends/family get this? Why doesn't anyone understand how hard this can be? Why can't people make more of an effort to support me? Why does "health food" have to be so expensive when it's all I can eat? Why won't my insurance company cover this medication/formula I need so badly? Sound familiar?

You may direct this anger towards family, friends, yourself, co-workers, medical staff, you pick. This is why it is so important to communicate with people so that they understand where you are coming from. This is also the time when you need to remember to stop, breathe, think, and then speak. There is nothing worse than adding fuel to a fire by adding your own spiteful words and anger. Your family is going through this as well, so remember that they are going through their own emotions and trying to support you the best way they know how. It may not be the way you think it should be done, but it is the best they can do. If that means you secretly want your significant other to make dinner one night, but she is scared to so she offers to walk the dog instead, then you need to accept that, breathe, and then say "thank you". You know what it is like to receive a guilt trip, try not to give any.

3   *Bargaining* – this is where you start to try to regain some control in your life. This is also where if you are going to "cheat" you are most likely to do it. You may think that you have been feeling really well lately, so maybe it isn't as bad as the doctors said it was. Maybe you could tolerate a small piece of fried chicken without your IBS flaring up, so you give it a try. This is when lessons are learned the hard way. Eventually you will learn, hopefully sooner than later, that "snitching" just isn't worth it. The damage done to your body, the way you feel, and the potential complications, just aren't worth that 30 seconds of instant gratification – trust me! If you do stray, accept it and move on. Stressing over it and feeling guilty will not do you any good. I just hope that you learn something from it, because if you did, then it wasn't a bad thing.

You may also try alternative/complimentary treatments at this stage. You may have heard about an herb that helps with inflammation in the colon – it worked wonders for your "friends cousin" so it should work for me. My strongest suggestion here, is if you are going to try some alternative/complimentary therapies, make sure you are working with a certified person in that field and that your attending physician is aware of it. Some won't affect medications like massage, but homeopathy, herbology and fad "diets" definitely can for example.

4   *Depression* – this is when you think, "this is my life and it kinda sucks". You miss going out for wings and beer with your friends on Thursday. You miss that your kids will never go to the county fair and stuff themselves full of mini donuts, corn dogs and candy. You wish that you and your family could just go out for a regular dinner without all the hassle.

You will always have these moments throughout your journey. But they will get less frequent and they will take less time to recover from. Taking time every day to take stock of what is *really* important in your life will help you through this stage, and the moments that will inevitably pop up. I still get these moments after 11 years of living with food restrictions; don't think for a moment that I don't. But, I am able to deal with them much better now and it has been years since I have cried in a grocery store!

5   *Acceptance* – "ok, I can do this". That is the best way to sum this phase up. You know what recipes work, you know what medical procedures need to be done, you know what medication, if any, needs to be taken when, you know how to go to social functions and not stress every moment, and most importantly, you know how to manage little things that pop up. You have the confidence in yourself, and those around you, to carry on living your life. You know where to go for help and support by now and you know how to advocate for yourself or your loved

one. By now, you don't obsess over not being able to eat certain foods; you are able to fully enjoy the ones you can.

The emotional roller coaster that you will be going on is different for everyone. Some may breeze through real easy; others may get stuck in one phase. If you notice that you or a loved one is having a difficult time managing or dealing with their food restrictions, there are professionals out there that can help. Even if you are a parent of a child going through the restrictions, there is a lot for you to deal with as well. There is no shame in talking with a counsellor or a psychologist, or other professional that can help you through. That is what they are there for. Your doctor may be able to refer you to one that deals with gastroenterology patients specifically. You do not need to go through this alone, so please don't. It only makes it harder on you and those around you. Reach out to friends and family. Search out support groups. Create a support group if there isn't one in your area. Go online and find people to connect with. If you feel there is no one out there, I am always here. Reach out to me, and I will help the best I can.

CHAPTER SIX

Proper Nutrition and Eating Strategies

Now to get into the fun stuff, what to eat to maintain your health. I want to emphasize that this is a general discussion on nutrition and I can offer suggestions, but each individual is their own person with their own diagnosis (or multiple diagnosis) and their own circumstances with their own medication list. This is why I highly suggest working with someone who is able to work with you specifically knowing your own health history. That being said, use this as a guide to get you started or supplement what you have already been told. Feel free to reach out if you have questions, you do not need to go through this alone, so there is no need to try. Trying on your own won't make you a saint, won't cure the problem, nor will it be less time consuming. It will be stressful. Trust me, I was there.

Because my daughter was diagnosed with her disease at such an early age when the medical community was just learning about the disease she had, we didn't have the support that is available now. Even when my son was born, there was a little more information available but not much. I still giggle when we see our team at the local Children's Hospital because our dietician still thanks me for coming in and teaching her something new to pass on to her other patients, or letting her taste a cookie that is made only with rice and apple products. While I love sharing this information, I sometimes wish it didn't take me years of experimenting and enormous amounts of thought over "what to feed my kids".

There are whole books dedicated to each one of these diseases/disorders and how to get and maintain proper nutrition, and I am going to just touch on each one to give you an overview. If you want more information, please go seek it out. Again, Chapter 9 provides you with a list of resources that you can go to. You can also reach out to your medical team, me, your family, or anyone else you feel will be able to give you the information you need.

There are a few basic things that need to be remembered regardless of your diagnosis about nutrition.

- Ensure you get enough water every day. A good rule of thumb is men need about 3.7 L/day and women need 2.7 L/day. Children need between 1.3 L and 2.4 L/day. Of course, please remember that there is water in the food you eat, the juices you consume, etc. You also need to equate your activity level into this. If you are more active, you should drink more water. And remember, our bodies play a trick on us; quite often we will misread the "thirsty" cue as a "hungry" cue.

- Fibre. Fibre. And fibre. For the general population, this needs to be taken in on a daily basis. Obviously for some of you out there, fibre can be an unpleasant thought. Regardless, please follow the guidelines for your own particular case and ensure you are getting enough quality fibre in your diet. This not only helps with bowel function but is also helpful in preventing/treating obesity and cardiovascular disease. Good sources of fibre are fruits, vegetables, legumes and whole grains.

- Fat is not your enemy, unless you have your gallbladder removed, then they can be. We need fats in our diets to ensure our bodies work properly. What we don't need are saturated and transfats, or too much of any type of fat. Generally speaking, the recommended amount of fat we need to consume daily is 20% - 35% of our daily intake. I personally believe that is a little high. I recommend to my clients that they consume 15% - 25% of their daily intake as fats – *good* fats. Fats found in naturally occurring plant sources such as nuts, seeds, fruits (olives, avocados, coconut, etc).

- Carbohydrates are sugars found in food. Most people think of them as your breads, pastas, etc, but they also include fruits and vegetables. It is important to get enough carbohydrates in your diet, diabetic or not. The trick is choosing quality carbohydrates such as whole grains, fruits and vegetables. Before you eat something you should think to yourself, "Is this cookie more or less nutritious than this mango?" The answer should be obvious, and so should your choice. But then there is the whole debate in your head about wanting that cookie instead, blah, blah, blah, and that is not the scope of this book *wink*.

- Protein is extremely important, and we need to make sure we all get enough, whether it is from animal sources or not. Vegans and vegetarians are able to get enough protein if they plan correctly. PKU patients are able to get their amino acids (building blocks of proteins) from specialized formula. Try to choose lean meats without visible fat (skin, marbling in a steak, etc).

Allergies

Depending on your allergy, you may need to completely eliminate one or more foods from your diet. If you need to do this, you need to ensure that some of the nutrients found in those foods are eaten in other foods. Depending on how well you do this you may or may not need to take a multivitamin. We are so lucky now because there are so many alternatives to cow's milk out there such as soy cheese, rice ice cream, almond puddings, etc. You will become a pro a reading labels and finding out the products you like/dislike. But, still do your best to ensure that you do not become deficient in a vitamin or mineral that is required for proper health/growth.

Here is a quick breakdown of the top 8 foods that people are allergic to, the nutrients in them, and other food sources to replace those nutrients.

Allergenic Food	Main Nutrients in that Food	Other Sources
Milk (cow's milk protein) and milk products (cheese, yogurt, etc)	Calcium; protein; vitamin D and Vitamin B12	Milk substitutes (soy, rice, almond, etc); broccoli; spinach; fortified foods; salmon; meat; fish; nuts
Peanuts	Biotin; copper; manganese; vitamin B3; folate; vitamin E	Mushrooms; egg yolks; avocados; organ meats; leafy vegetables; tomatoes; fortified/enriched foods
Tree Nuts	Fatty acids; fibre; vitamin E; folic acid; calcium; potassium	Fish; whole grains; fruits; vegetables; tomatoes; spinach; avocados; fortified/enriched foods

Allergenic Food	Main Nutrients in that Food	Other Sources
Fish	Protein; fatty acids; calcium; vitamin D; vitamin B6; Niacin	Lean meats; avocados; olives; dairy products; leafy green vegetables; tomatoes; chickpeas; potatoes; bananas
Shellfish	Protein; vitamin B12; zinc; choline	Lean meats; legumes; eggs; liver; fortified/enriched foods; cottage cheese;
Eggs	Protein; biotin; choline; iron; vitamin A; vitamin D; vitamin E; vitamin B12;	Lean meats; legumes; liver; carrots; sweet potato; fish; fortified milk and cereals; nuts; seeds; spinach
Wheat	Fibre; iron; manganese; niacin; phosphorous; magnesium	Fruits and vegetables; other whole grains (rice, quinoa, corn; millet; buckwheat, etc)
Soy	Protein; fat; calcium; iron	Lean meats; milk products; legumes

If you or your loved one is diagnosed with one or two allergies, it really isn't that difficult to manage once you learn the substitutions you need to make and learn how to read labels. Yes it seems very overwhelming, as does any new diagnosis. But learning how to bake with soy milk versus cow's milk is an easy step to take, or realizing that you need to choose peanut free treats over the peanut butter cups you used to have, can be managed. There are so many options out there in the grocery stores that after you spend some time learning how to grocery shop again, then it will become easier. Just remember to *read every label*.

Celiac Disease

Oh the options you have now compared to ten years ago! There are gluten free cookies, breads, muffins, pizzas, and even beer available now, even in restaurants. No more are the days of eating rice and vegetables for every meal. Once you get used to reading labels and trying different gluten free products (there are good and bad, and then really bad) then you will have a handle on what you can eat. Remember to check the ingredients on processed foods and condiments because quite often they will have gluten in them as well.

The trick is, after you are diagnosed work with a dietician/nutritionist to figure out what nutrients are lacking in your diet currently. I would also recommend your doctor run a blood test to see how your current nutrition status is; find out what vitamins/minerals are deficient in you because remember, one of the symptoms of Celiac Disease is the inability to absorb nutrients due to the damaged villi in your intestine. Once you have figured out what your current status is, it is time to start replacing those vitamins and minerals and build your health back up.

I wish I could simply state, "eat gluten free whole grains and you are good to go". Unfortunately, I can't because of the variables that exist in each case such as the severity of the damage to the villi, how long it has been undiagnosed, current food intake, and associated problems. But I can assure you that once you understand what is going on, accept that you will be on this new path of eating for the rest of your life, and learn (sometimes the hard way) that cheating really isn't worth it, and then you'll be healthy and feeling great!

One misconception people have, unfortunately, is that if it is gluten free it is healthy. Nope. Often people with Celiac Disease are so excited that they can eat a gluten free cookie that tastes good, that they will forget basic nutrition and gorge themselves on those cookies because they haven't been able to for so long. It is sometimes hard to remember that eating healthy is still just as important. 2500 calories equals one pound. If you eat an extra 357 calories in a day over and above what your body needs, you will put on 1 pound in a week. That's only about 5 extra gluten free cookies a day, above what you need. For someone who hasn't enjoyed a good cookie in years, and can eat a whole package in one sitting, that math isn't going to add up well on your waistline.

Crohn's/Colitis

Because these two diseases are so individualized and can change over time, it is very important to work with a nutrition-ist/dietician to ensure that you are properly managing it. There is not one particular food that is problematic, nor is there one food that will fix everything. I did discuss earlier what to do nutritionally during a flare up, and depending on what is going on where, your strategy for nutrition will change. A well balanced diet, focussing on healthy eating strategies, is incredibly important for these patients.

There are a variety of factors that can affect your nutrition, whether it is your appetite level, medication, or inflammation levels. All of these can affect how many nutrients you are absorbing. So, what you chose to eat is very important because your body will get the nutrition it requires from healthy foods, not from junk food. And in those people who just can't eat, or don't want to, a meal replacement drink is always an option for you. The last thing you want to do is get malnourished and add to your troubles.

Depending on your health status, your fibre intake may need to be changed. This is where working with your medical team is important. If you are having severe inflammation, adding unsolu-able fibre to your diet is only going to aggravate your intestine. If you have severe diarrhea, then adding fibre is a good idea. So again, it is important to get that individualized care from your team.

Here are some general tips for Crohn's and Colitis patients:

- Ensure you get enough fluids
- Avoid caffeine and fruit juices
- Keep meals small and frequent
- Keep a food journal to see what aggravates your symptoms

Diabetes

I really cannot emphasize enough how important it is to establish a good rapport with your team, stay on top of your glucose levels, and take your insulin if required. If you are able to control your diabetes with diet alone – do it, because if you don't then it may progress to the point where you need to take insulin daily. And I don't know about you, but if I had the option of not sticking a needle in me, and sticking a needle in me, I would choose the first option (that is why I didn't become a doctor or nurse... I hate needles!)

Maintaining proper nutrition for Diabetics is relatively easy, once you learn how to use the Glycemic Index/Load and learn how to control your glucose levels. In fact, following a Diabetic Diet is one of the healthier eating strategies out there because it focuses on portion control, lots of fresh fruit and veggies, lean meats, reduced sugar consumption and frequent snacks. The snacking part is really important for Diabetics and is often over looked. The reason for frequent snacks is to ensure that your glucose levels stay at a constant, without spikes or falls. If you have a little something every 2 or 3 hours, then your levels should stay relatively stable, accounting for the fact that that little something is not simple carbohydrate or sugar laden.

There are a few special considerations that Diabetics should take into account:

- Maintain a stable weight rather than having it go up and down; gradually lose weight if overweight
- If chronic kidney disease is present, monitor your protein intake
- Take a supplement if required to achieve adequate vitamin and mineral intake
- Pay attention to your physical and mental status as well, because those may be indicative of symptoms arising associated with uncontrolled Diabetes
- Spend some time planning your meals and being prepared
- Chromium and magnesium deficiencies can affect how the body uses insulin
- Dietary plans should focus on heart disease reduction as well as blood glucose management

(38)

Diverticulitis

This one sounds easier than it is – avoid small seeds and nuts. But have you actually thought about all the foods that contain small seeds? Strawberries, kiwis, raspberries, sesame seeds, grapes, and the list goes on. The good news is, most of the vitamins and minerals that are found in those nuts and seeds, are found elsewhere and as long as you eat a healthy, varied diet you should be ok. Currently, the jury is out about the amount of fibre for diverticulitis. Some say it should be a low fibre diet; others are starting to say that a regular fibre diet is fine. My personal opinion is to get enough different types of fibre in your diet and monitor your symptoms with a food journal. I also tend to lean towards avoiding smaller seeds and nuts. Of course, each person is different, so ensure you work with your current medical team and follow their recommendations.

Eosinophilic Gastrointestinal Disorders

You want to talk about nutritional information and needing your team, you read this section! The severity of this disorder can be as simple as avoiding one or two foods, or as complicated as taking medication and having to be tube fed an elemental formula. I really cannot say what you can and cannot eat. Nor can I give you some general guidelines because each case is so individualized. Some people need to avoid milk; others milk and soy; yet others may need to avoid cinnamon. The combination of possibilities is enormous! But, I can say that this disorder is closely linked with allergies and if you know that you are allergic to anything (in the clinical sense), then definitely avoid it. I don't even want to recommend taking a multivitamin to any of you without warning you to check the ingredients. I have yet to find a safe multivitamin for my kids.

Definitely work with your medical team. As mentioned earlier, you need to really build this trust and respect, because this is an ongoing disorder that can change over time. A nutritionist/dietician is critical to work with. He or she will find out what vitamins/minerals may be lacking and be able to provide you with alternative sources that are safe for your particular case. And, if you are severe enough to warrant an amino acid based formula, they will be instrumental in helping you get that.

Because food is such a social aspect, if you suffer from EGID then my suggestion here would be to get as much variety as you can with the limited foods you may have. For example, if you can have apples then dehydrate them, eat them raw, bake them, BBQ them, juice them, make apple sauce, put them in the pancakes or muffins you can bake, grind up dehydrated apples in a new coffee grinder to use as a "sugar" on things, peel them, and do whatever else you can. Let your imagination sore and you will find lots of ways to enjoy one single food. If you are unable to eat meats, beans, and legumes as your regular source of protein, find other alternatives to protein and use them. For example, I can purchase a rice protein powder and I put in a scoop into the basmati rice I make to bump up the protein levels in it. It is still just rice, but a little more nutritional.

If you do require an amino acid formula, remember that you can use it in other methods other than just via tube feed or drinking orally. I always put a scoop of the powder into everything I make for the kids. Their safe pancakes, meatloaf, cookies, etc. Adding a scoop doesn't hurt and can only add nutrition where it is needed. But if you do decide to do this be careful because adding too much will really change the regular taste of it and it might not be as enjoyable.

Irritable Bowel Syndrome

Google® this topic and you will find so many different suggestions on what to eat, what not to eat, what supplements to take, and how to manage your diet that you will get overwhelmed and confused. Again, every person has their own triggers and their own emotions, and stress is a very common trigger for IBS. I remember years ago my daughters' previous gastroenterologist and I were talking about IBS and he asked me, "When you think about something that really angers you, or upsets you, doesn't your stomach get upset and grumble a bit? Now imagine your stomach and intestines are already unhappy – wouldn't that make it worse?" Simple logic is sometimes the best. That being said, there are some things you can do to help keep your tummy happy:

- Manage your stress levels. Some ways to do this is to get regular exercise, take 5 minutes out a day for yourself and just be quiet, learn different stress management techniques.

- Avoid caffeine

- Find out what your trigger foods are by keeping a food diary

- You may benefit from an elimination diet to help you discover your food triggers if you are severe with your IBS, if this is the case, make sure you are working with a dietician/nutritionist to ensure that you are doing this in a healthy manner and not causing more problems.

- Fibre. Yes, no or maybe? Well, this depends on your own particular case. Sometimes people with IBS do well on a small amount of insoluble fibre, others need more. Again, only your experience will tell you.

- Try to eat meals at the same time to get your body used to a regular schedule. Also, keep them small and frequent.

- Eat your meals slowly, and relaxed. Anybody who rushes through their meal will get a tummy ache and feel bloated, let along someone with IBS.

- Keep a water bottle with you at all times and drink water throughout the day. First of all, if you have diarrhea, you need to replenish lost fluids. If you have constipation, the water will help with that. If you get tired of plain water, add in some fresh fruit to it to flavour it – I personally love lemon, watermelon or strawberries in my water.

Intolerances

This one is easy to say, hard to do. If it bugs you don't eat it. That being said, if you have lactose intolerance, you are missing the enzyme in your digestive system to digest the lactose, and thankfully there are enzyme supplements you can take prior to eating lactose that can help. In regards to other foods, try to avoid them.

There are lots of causes for food intolerances, and that is beyond the scope of this discussion. Regardless of what causes your intolerance, you will be your own expert in what foods bother you and what foods don't. This is where a food diary can come in really handy. And not just for a few days. Keep track of what you eat, what your symptoms are and when they happen for at least a week in my opinion; keeping in mind that it may take a few days for symptoms to show up with an intolerance. And symptoms can be extremely varied, as mentioned previously.

People with intolerances need to really listen to their body. The trick is, sometimes we feel so bad for so long, that we think it is normal. For this reason, often I recommend to my clients to go on a minor elimination diet avoiding processed food, gluten, and milk, all the while eating plenty of fresh fruit, veggies and whole grains for a couple weeks to get their bodies into a state of feeling well. Then we introduce foods again to see if symptoms arise. Food diaries – a food intolerant person's bible!

PKU

A lifelong diet of reducing intake of the amino acid phenylalanine to the minimum amount needed, which essentially means reducing "normal" protein intake by 80% is necessary, this means avoiding very protein rich foods such as eggs, meats, dairy products, peanuts, and soy products. It may go against what society sees as healthy, but eating foods high in fat and sugars, and low in natural proteins, are safe for people with PKU.

People who have PKU need to work extremely close with their medical team to ensure that adequate nutrition is achieved, mainly through specialized formulas and foods that are designed for patients with PKU. These foods provide the protein required for the patient, while eliminating the amino acid phenylalanine.

The key concept to remember with PKU patients is low protein. Protein is found in many foods, including grains, cereals, etc. So foods need to be closely monitored to ensure that optimum health is achieved and maintained.

Summary

I realize that many of you are probably looking for more detail on how to achieve/maintain nutrition for your own particular case. I understand. I remember when I was going through the initial stages of learning how to feed my children I wanted someone to tell me, "feed her/him this and all will be OK."

Unfortunately, as a professional, I am unable to do that in this book because each case is so individual and specific that I don't want to steer anyone the wrong way. But, as a parent I completely understand where you are coming from! You just want someone to tell you what to do and how to do it because your brain in is overload. This is where I urge you to reach out and work with a nutritionist, dietician, somebody. Unfortunately, your physician is a very busy person and they can give you guidelines and the basics, but they have hundreds of kids to treat, not just yours. So, when you reach out to a nutritionist/dietician they usually are able to take the extra time needed to work with you a little closer and specifically.

Please be patient and understanding. This is a process with a lot of trial and error. If you are at all concerned about the nutritional status of yourself or loved one, check into whether or not taking a high quality multivitamin is safe. Or look into safe meal replacements that provide full nutrition and see if that is an option for you. There are options out there. There are people who can help you. Reach out to them because you will only add to your already existent stress level if you try to do this alone.

CHAPTER SEVEN

Complimentary Therapies

Some people call them alternative therapies, some people call them complimentary, and others call them wastes of time. I personally like to think of these treatments/therapies as complimentary, meaning they work together along with traditional Western medical treatments. Alternative therapies generally imply that they are used in place of Western medical practices. It is not secret that I firmly believe in working with your medical team. Personally, I am 100% sure that my children would not be as healthy as they are without my medical team so I am never going to discount working with them. But, I also believe there are many things you can do to supplement, or work with, the care and treatment that is being provided by your medical team.

What may work for one person, may not work for another. For example, my mom responds very well to Reiki, where as my husband thinks it is hogwash, yet he swears by acupuncture. If you are interested in learning about or trying some complimentary treatments, as I mentioned previously, please ensure that you are being treated by a certified professional and that your regular physician is aware of it. Some physicians embrace the practice of using complimentary therapies, others don't. Take their opinions to heart, make informed decisions, and proceed with figuring out that works best for you and your health. You are the one ultimately responsible for your health, from deciding whether or not to "cheat", to whether or not you think a certain therapy is the best choice for you.

I will go over some of the common complimentary therapies that are out there, list their theory, pros and cons, and hopefully help you on your way to making a more informed decision.

Accupressure/Accupuncture

Acupressure is Acupuncture without the tiny needles. They both follow the same belief and guidelines so I will address them as one here. Acupuncture is based on the ancient Chinese belief that we all have *chi*, or life energy that flows through us and every living thing. This energy flows through our body via *meridians* which are connected to specific organs. When we are healthy and there are no problems, our energy is thought to be flowing freely without obstruction. But when we have a disease or illness, the belief is that the flow of energy is blocked going to that particular area and needs to be released or unblocked. Kind of like a hose. If there is nothing blocking the hose, then water flows freely and everything work fine. But if there is a small kink in that hose, water runs slower taking longer to nourish the garden you are trying to water. If that hose is completely blocked, then you are unable to water that garden and it will not grow properly. Unblock the hose, water flows freely, then the garden can grow.

Because the belief is in releasing energy blocks, there are no contradictions with any medications or procedures your medical doctor may be using. There may be some discomfort when the tiny needles for acupuncture are placed, kind of like when you prick yourself with a needle when you are sewing. But after the needle is inserted, you hardly realize there is anything there. With acupressure, the practitioner will just press on certain points and that may cause slight discomfort, but is immediately gone when the pressure is released. Some practitioners will suggest herbal remedies, exercises, and possibly lifestyle changes. If herbal remedies are being suggested, ensure that you are fully aware, and inform your doctor, of any herbs you are taking and what possible contradictions may occur. In regards to exercises and lifestyle changes, as long as it is for the best I see no reason to worry.

Aromatherapy

Aromatherapists use essential oils to enhance a person's wellbeing, whether physical or mental. The theory goes that when you inhale the essential oil, it triggers your olfactory system which in turns triggers a part of your brain to react to that smell, causing an emotional response. It can even be claimed by some that physical ailments can be lessened or helped in response to this reaction. It kind of makes sense. Scientists have determined recently that the pleasure center in women's brains (the center that responds when you eat chocolate, laugh, etc), light up when they smell the aroma of a newborn baby (whether or not they had just given birth). Think about how you feel when you smell fresh cut grass, or fresh roses, or your favourite cologne... you smile or feel happy, or something. That smell triggers a physiological and/or emotional response in us. The same premise exists for aromatherapy.

When using essential oils, highly concentrated distilled oils of plants, precautions do need to be taken. Often one or two drops is all you need in a whole diffuser to achieve the effect. The oils are extremely potent and some can actually harm you if put directly on your skin or ingested. When using essential oils for the skin, quite often a few drops of the oil is mixed in with another carrier oil such as olive oil, jojoba oil, etc. Massage therapists sometimes add a few drops of essential oil to their massage oil to help create a relaxing atmosphere for their client.

My personal view on aromatherapy is simple. If it works, great; if it doesn't then your house smells of lavender naturally instead of with a synthetic spray. As long as you are using them safely, then I don't see any harm in trying. Talk to a registered aromatherapist and ensure you are fully informed and using them safely. There are many companies/people out there that will promise you the moon or perfect health, but like the adage said, "buyers beware". Like I said, if nothing else it may help you feel relaxed, happy, or whatever. Our bodies are so interconnected that our emotions can affect us physically, so if it helps you relax, if nothing else, than what harm is it in trying?

Ayurvedic Remedies

Ayurvedic medicine uses meditation, herbs, yoga, mental visualization, breathing exercises, exercise, diet, color therapy, aromatherapy, sound therapy and massage to treat an illness and maintain health. It is one of the oldest forms of medicine in the world and works on the body as a whole, rather than its individual parts. According to this practice, there are three energies (doshas) that work together in the body: vata (from ether and air), pitta (from fire and water), and kapha (from water and earth). One type of dosha is usually dominated over the other ones in any individual and when your doshas are out of balance, then illness occurs. By using herbs and the other modalities listed above, the practitioner will get your body back into balance and then your body should start healing itself. Because there are so many different methods that can be used to bring your body back into balance between the three doshas, I would recommend that you practice caution when it comes to each individual practice and use your discretion. Obviously some practices like color therapy and sound therapy you don't need to worry about too much, but be aware when it comes to herbs and anything you are taking orally; these may counteract with medications you may be taking.

Chinese Medicine

Another really old form of medicine, Chinese Medicine, mainly aims at preventing disease, rather than treating it. One of the main tenants of Chinese medicine is to make the necessary lifestyle changes to obtain balance in the body. If your body is out of balance, then various treatments may be used to get your body back into balance, where health will then flourish. With balance, your own energy, or chi, is flowing correctly and you have a equilibrium of yin and yang, which are present in everybody and everything. Some earth elements are classified as yin, some are classified as yang; same with foods, bodily function and herbs. Chinese Medical practitioners will use certain herbs, foods, massage practices, and acupuncture/acupressure to bring your body back into balance.

Some Chinese Medicine herbs can be extremely potent, and I highly suggest that if you are looking at this modality, seek out a qualified practitioner. Many over the counter Chinese medicines are not really traditional and are not always pure – simply put they are the western world's way of cashing in on a current trend. If you are truly interested, do your homework and be aware. Also, let your primary physician know so that any medications won't be contradicted.

Chiropractic

Chiropractic care operates on the theory that signals travel from the brain down our spinal cord to various organs in our body. If the spine is out of alignment, then the signals are unable to travel freely and then pain and other disorders may arise. Therefore, chiropractors will adjust the spine to allow signals to flow normally and then the body will be able to heal itself and the pain and discomfort should lessen. Chiropractors also help with the pain of physical spinal misalignment (lower back pain, neck pain, ribs misaligned, etc). They definitely serve their purpose and have their place in the health care system.

As with any modality, if you feel uncomfortable with anything your chiropractor is doing, let them know. Different chiropractors use different methods to help align the spine. Some are very "hands on" and physically manipulate your spine, while other will use a small tool called an "adjuster" to gently help the vertebras move. You need to openly communicate with your chiropractor to suit your comfort level. For example, as a young teenager, I had a tobogganing accident that resulted in a compound fracture of my neck and a broken tailbone. As a result, I still have some problems with my neck today and recently had to see a chiropractor. Because of my neck injury (and resulting herniated disks) I am very hesitant to let anyone manipulate my neck, unless they use the "clicky thingy" (adjuster). I was upfront and open about this and the chiropractor thanked me for indicating this before the session began because he is very "hands on" and rarely uses it. If I hadn't been open about that, the whole experience would have been very different and I wouldn't have gotten the much needed relief I needed.

Colon Cleansing

The theory with colon cleansing is that gunk left in the colon builds up toxins that will affect your whole body, showing up as symptoms such as allergic reactions, irritability, gastrointestinal problems, tiredness and even depression. According to colonic practitioners, if you cleanse the colon of all this debris, and clear the toxins from your body, then you should be on the path to recovery.

The way to perform a colon cleanse varies according to individual practitioners, but the general process is going on a fast for a few days, using herbs and fibre supplements to help get rid of the toxins in your body, then slowly reintroduce foods into your diet starting with only raw foods, then a set amount of cooked foods along with the raw, etc. Sometimes enemas or colonics (a treatment that flushes the colon) will be used as well.

For anybody who has gastrointestinal issues, I urge you to be careful, especially if using enemas or colonics. Think about it, if your colon is damaged already, using a method that could potentially cause more harm is not a good idea. But, keeping your body/colon as "clean" as possible by eating a lot of raw foods and ensuring you get enough fibre is a good idea. But if you are in a flare up with your Colitis, eating a lot of unsoluable fibre could aggravate your symptoms. So, if you are considering this, please make sure you are working with a certified practitioner, nutritionist, and definitely let your physician know.

Guided Imagery

This process works on the premise that positive thoughts will enhance your immune system function and will help reduce stress. Basically, think of a time when you were in a miserable mood and everything just seemed to go wrong and you felt absolutely "yucky". Then think of another time when you were having a terrific day, felt great, and everything was going well. The theory is, that if you are able to replace your negative thoughts/feelings with positive ones, then you will feel better physically and emotionally.

So for example, if a person had Celiac Disease and their villi were still damaged from recent gluten exposure, then that person could picture the villi lifting up, moving freely, and absorbing the nutrients they need to absorb. This doesn't mean that you can go eat a fresh croissant then imagine yourself better. What it does mean is that you can imagine yourself healthy and you may just feel a little better. By no means is this to replace medical advice, but what harm can it do to sit down and imagine your body absorbing the nutrients it requires to help repair any damage and maintain optimum health.

Homeopathy

Homeopathy is based on the premise that the body has a natural ability to heal itself and symptoms are seen as the body's way to protect itself from disease. With this train of thought, homeopathic practitioners give the individual small amounts of what is causing the symptom to aid the body in healing itself. So, for example, if you were allergic to eggs and saw a homeopathic practitioner to help you, he/she would give you minute amounts of egg, along with other homeopathic remedies, to help the body heal itself from that allergy. The practitioner treats the person as a whole, not just the symptom. So if our individual with the egg allergy is given remedies A, B, and C another person with an egg allergy would be given remedies D, E and F because those are those ones that will work for that individual person.

You can purchase homeopathic remedies at many health food stores and even some pharmacies. The amounts of active ingredient in the remedies are very small so theoretically, there should be no contradiction with any current medication that you are taking. That being said, I would still search out a qualified practitioner to work with. Because homeopathy works when the whole person is treated individually and not just treating a specific symptom you have, you need a practitioner who has specialized training. Some naturopaths and other practitioners are qualified to work with homeopathy, so they may suggest using this as part of their treatment plan with you.

Massage

Ahhh, massage! What feels better than having your sore muscles eased by a great massage? But, there other benefits to massage than just easing sore muscles. Massage works by manipulating muscles and soft tissues in your body promoting relaxation, increased circulation of the blood and lymphatic systems, and helping drain away toxins that have built up in these tissues as well. In particular for people with gastrointestinal discomfort, it can help there too. For example, if you are constipated, massaging the abdomen in a clockwise motion can help move things along (if you go counter clockwise though, you will be pushing the fecal matter further up into your colon).

Gentle massages you can do on your own, on a loved one, or by a registered massage therapist. There are different types of massage, and depending on your needs and comfort level, you may have a preference for one over another. Here is a short list of some of the different types of massage:

- Deep Tissue Massage – deeper pressure is applied to get further into the tissues to help release chronic tension and muscle problems.

- Esalen Massage – this technique works on the whole person to greatly relax the person by using repetitive, rhythmic motions.

- Neuromuscular Massage – this is a form of deep tissue massage that also works with various trigger points to release pressure and increase blood flow.

- Reflexology – this form of massage works mainly on your feet, but sometimes on your hands and other areas, and applies pressure to certain points to open a channel of energy to flow.

- Rolfing – this method works on the tissues that connect your muscles to your bones to bring your body back into alignment, and therefore bringing your body into balance.

- Shiatsu – this is an Oriental technique that uses acupressure points, stroking, tapping, stretching and kneading as part of the session.

- Sports Massage – not only is deep tissue massage used by sports massage therapist, but also stretching and kneading.
- Swedish Massage – this is a relaxation type of massage that uses gentle motions along with tapping and kneading.

As with any complimentary therapy, you need to be comfortable and honest with your massage therapist. I honestly do not see an issue with anybody who is required to restrict their foods to avoid seeing a massage therapist, but as you can see there are many different types of massage to choose from. You just need to know what you want the massage for, and then find a qualified person to do it for you. Or, as I mentioned before, you can massage yourself or a loved one. Keep the lines of communication open and if for some reason you are ever uncomfortable (physically or emotionally) let your massage therapist know.

One word of caution; massage therapists use massage oils and sometimes add essential oils to them. If you have any allergies, be sure to let them know. For example, when I asked my massage therapist to work on my daughter, I provided her with rice oil to use so that she didn't create an allergic reaction.

Meditation

Meditation is a form of just "being" and in today's society of go, go, go, it is hard to do that. Most people when they think of meditation they think of someone sitting on the floor, in a convoluted sitting position, chanting to themselves. Not true. Meditation in its' basic form is just a way to quiet the mind and relax. Some people do meditate in the middle of the floor, sitting and chanting. Others are able to quiet the mind by sitting on the lawn tractor cutting the grass, like my mother.

Yet others are able to just sit and stare at nothing, while others will picture an image in their mind and focus on that or a sound.

Meditation offers no harm if you practice it. If nothing else it will make you sit down and take a few moments out of your day to just let your thoughts come and go. You have nothing to lose in trying meditation.

Reiki

Reiki is a form of energy healing that works on the premise that everyone has 7 major chakras and then some minor chakras. If one or more of these chakras becomes blocked then illness/disease occurs. The Reiki practitioner will channel energy through them to you via their hands to help unblock these chakras and place their hands either directly on you or just above you. They may also employ crystals as part of their session based on the belief that the crystals themselves hold a particular energy that may help you.

Reiki works on the person as a whole and will go to where it is needed most, regardless of what you or the practitioner thinks. So for example, if you feel that constipation is the main issue that you need to have worked on, the practitioner will work on your whole body and you may feel it in your throat more than in your abdomen. Or, you may not physically feel anything, yet emotionally feel a difference (sad, happy, energized, etc). If nothing else, Reiki is generally very relaxing and poses no risk to you regardless of the disease/disorder you have.

Be prepared though to not have what you want to feel/happen to happen, because as much as the practitioner wants to help you, the Reiki energy may go to an issue that is more pressing than the physical ailment you are suffering from. The theory is that problems arise in a spiritual/emotional level and then manifest themselves as physical issues. So that constipation issue you may have may not be as important to treat as the emotional issue that may have affected you prior.

Summary

Regardless of whether or not you want to look into complimentary therapies, I want to impress one string of commonality that runs through a lot of these modalities – stress reduction. I highly suggest that each of you, especially those of you who are caring for a person with food restrictions, find some avenue to help you reduce your stress levels. It took me a long time to figure this out and to accept the fact that if I didn't look after myself, then how could I look after my family. My husband was integral in teaching me that it is OK to indulge in myself every once in a while to ensure that I don't get too stressed out, which in turn would affect my health.

A great analogy was given to me about how stress affects each person and those around them. Imagine you are holding a can of pop. Each time something happens that makes you feel stressed, shake that can of pop. So, you are running late in the morning. Shake. Then your child tells you that it is cupcake day at school today and you didn't have a chance to make safe cupcakes. Shake. Then as you walk out the door, your tire is flat. Shake. You get the idea. Now, who wants to open that can of pop? If you do, not only will you, but those around you, get sprayed with sugary, sticky pop. If you manage the stress, then that can of pop can't explode.

(17)

CHAPTER EIGHT

My Own Two Cents

You may be thinking, "Why is she writing this chapter when this whole book is her own two cents?" Easy, these are my after thoughts that don't quite fit easily into any of the chapters that are included. This chapter is my little bits of inspiration, wisdom, and professional experience that I hope will make this journey a little easier for you.

You may recall that my goal in writing this book is to help you get through this journey as unscathed as possible. There will always be people challenging you with, "one bite won't hurt," or "you look fine, how can you be that sick", or my favourite, "but there is only one egg in that cake batter" or whatever ammo they may have. Please remember that it is not that these people are trying to hurt you or offend you – they honestly just do not understand what is going on. Take this opportunity to teach them. Educate old Aunt Bess about Diabetes and what does happen if you eat that homemade candy she spent hours preparing. And be patient. Not everyone will "get it", just like I don't "get" physics. (Funny story, my husband and I knew each other in school and I had asked him multiple times to help me with my physics homework... and he now jokes that he finally got paid for that tutoring years later.)

Professionally, I am here to help anyone ensure that they get the proper nutrition they require. I am also here to help my clients through the struggles of dealing with food restrictions. I offer many tips to my clients that I would like to share with you so that you can ensure not only are you managing your food restrictions, but that you are as healthy as possible.

- If you can't pronounce it, you probably shouldn't eat it.

- Enjoy cooking at home – for a few reasons. First of all, you know exactly what the ingredients are, if there was cross-contamination of foods, and most importantly you get to discover the wonderful ways of using simple ingredients to make amazing meals. One thing I like to do is make presentation everything. Even though my kids' dinner consists of rice paper rolls filled with rice and apple slices, I arrange them beautifully in a circle on a plate with apple slices and apple butter in a pretty little dish in the center. Cut the pancakes into a heart shape for Valentine's Day, or a four-leaf clover for St. Patrick's Day. Don't you enjoy a beautiful dish presentation in a restaurant? Why not do it at home?!

- I do not recommend a vegetarian diet, a vegan diet, a low fat diet, a meat and potato diet, or a high protein/low carb diet. What I do recommend is to listen to your body, rec-ognize your symptoms and eat what makes you feel the best. For some that means vegetarian, others it means "meatless Monday", some it means meat and potatoes eve-ry night, yet for others it may mean a lot of protein. My husband has absolutely no food restrictions at all, yet he doesn't feel well after eating chicken. So we don't eat a lot of chicken. Listening to your body is hard. Because your body screams, "don't eat that!" yet your mind says, "oh but it is so good, one bite won't hurt!" Eventually you will learn that your body is an incredibly intelligent thing and it is giving you cues as to what works and what doesn't. It will make things a lot easier in the long run, if you listen, and obey, what your boy is telling you.

- Have you ever noticed that after you eat Chinese food or eat something from a fast food joint that you are hungry again in half an hour? There is a reason for this. Your body sends out hunger signals when it requires nutrition. If you aren't giving your body whole foods that provide proper nutrition, your body is going to say, "feed me, I need proper nutrition". When you eat processed foods your body is not able to get the nutrition it needs from it. If you eat lots of whole grains, fruits and vegetables for dinner, you won't get those hunger pains right after because your body is able to absorb the nutrients it requires. It may take a few days of eating this way before your body realizes that you are feeding it properly, but it will reward you.

- Don't mix up thirst cues for hunger cues. We often do this. If you start feeling hungry, have a glass of water first – especially if you just had a meal or snack. It might be your body is just thirsty.

- Remember why you are here. You are here to learn and grow as a person and spread joy and love to those around you. Sometimes we get so wrapped up in daily life and food management strategies that we forget that we are in this world to be us. We are here to enjoy our families and friends. We are here to learn lessons and teach other. We are here for a reason – even though we may not know what it is. I firmly believe that we are only given the challenges that we can handle, and that has gotten me through a lot of challenges. Try to figure out what makes you tick and re-member that. If you are a parent, try to stop for even a few minutes a day to enjoy your children – they are one of the reasons you are here.

- My husband taught me a very valuable lesson – it's OK to do things for you. Not only is it OK, it is necessary. This is a really hard lesson for some people to learn, especially if you are a parent of a child with massive food restrictions. After all, you are consumed with keeping your child healthy, isn't that the most important thing? Yes, but how are you going to take care of anybody else, be it child, spouse, friend, or extended family, if you are dead meat or unhealthy yourself. How are you going to spend the day cooking a weeks' worth of Diabetic meals for your father, if you are on the couch reeling in pain from an IBS flare up? Or how are you going to get up in the middle of the night with your child who is in so much pain they are crying because you forgot to take your own medication the night before and can't get out of bed due to your own pain? You *have* to take care of you – physically, emotionally, spiritually and mentally. Find your escape and allow yourself to go there once in a while. Find an exercise that you enjoy and do it. Find a peaceful place in your mind and go there to regroup and relax. Find something to challenge yourself with mentally. Your brain is a muscle that needs exercise as well...

- BREATHE! I took my kids to a ceramic shop once to paint some ceramics. I had made a mug with the saying, "we are not granted patience, just opportunities to practice it". My kids know that when I am having a cup of tea out of that mug to leave me alone until my tea is gone. It is my message to the world that I need to BREATHE right now, and you better let me, otherwise I will go "nuclear" as my husband so eloquently puts it. Dealing with severe or multiple food restrictions can be very stressful and consuming, so I strongly suggest you find your subtle message to those around you to leave you alone so you can BREATHE.

The final two cents I would like to leave you with is to trust yourself. If your gut (pardon the pun) is telling you something, then investigate further. You are the only one who knows you as well as you do. Better than your doctor, better than your family, and better than your friends. But, don't talk yourself into something that isn't there. We can all manage to talk ourselves into a tizzy, so we can all manage to talk ourselves out of one. And while we all have the best intentions, and we arm ourselves with knowledge, we need to remember that there may not always be a problem there. Even though you have chronic stomach pain, you may have stomach pain this time around due to a virus that you are sick with rather than a flare up of IBS.

I want each and every one of you to remember one thing that will get you through living with food restrictions; you are not alone and you are blessed. You may not see it now, but you are. Food restrictions are a blessing in disguise. You are forced to listen to your body and pay attention to minute details that many people simply over look. You are forced to have compassion and understanding beyond what other people may have. You are forced to become a lifelong learner. You are forced to become a better person. So remember to give thanks for everything, including your food restrictions.

CHAPTER NINE

Where to Go for More

In today's society, it is easy to get inundated with information and sensory overload. You can literally spend hours searching the internet for information on any topic that you want. Some of that information is credible, some isn't. I may be aging myself a little here, but when my daughter was an infant, I lived in a small town and we didn't have access to high speed internet, only the big cities did. So my hours of research were even more painful because I had to deal with dial up connections. Even then, I managed to find credible sources to take to my doctors at the time to help find a diagnosis for my daughter. Thankfully, things move a lot quicker now.

As wonderful as the internet is, and all that we can learn from different people and organizations, we still need to be careful to not self diagnose a problem and search so hard that we actually do find an answer that we want, even though it may not be correct. That being said, please do educate yourself with credible sources. I have compiled a list of resources for you to begin your own search. These sites are reputable, credible, and have my trust in them. They are categorized into separate diseases/disorders to make it even easier for you to find what you are looking for, or at least start. In the general health category, you can find information on all of the diseases/disorders and general gastrointestinal health. By no means is this comprehensive, and I am sure that there are many more wonderful websites out there that I have not included, but I wanted to keep this relatively short and sweet. This is a starting place for you and I'm sure you will find other great resources in your journey.

General Health

International Foundation for Functional Gastrointestinal Disorders
http://www.iffgd.org/

Canadian Digestive Health Foundation
http://www.cdhf.ca/en/home/

Patient UK
http://www.patient.co.uk/

Medline Plus
http://www.nlm.nih.gov/ medlineplus/medlineplus.html

Web MD
http://www.webmd.com/

Rare Disease
www.raredisease.org

Health Finder
www.healthfinder.gov

Kids Health
www.kidshealth.org

GI Kids
www.gikids.org

General Nutrition

Canada's Food Guide Tracker
http://www.hc-sc.gc.ca/fn-an/food-guide-aliment/track-suivi/index-eng.php

USDA Choose My Plate
www.choosemyplate.gove

Academy of Nutrition and Dietetics
www.eatright.org

Celiac

Celiac Support Association
http://www.csaceliacs.org

Canadian Celiac Association
http://www.celiac.ca/

National Foundation for Celiac Awareness
http://www.celiaccentral.org/support-groups/

Celiac.com
http://www.celiac.com/

Celiac Disease Foundation
http://celiac.org/

Gluten Intolerance Group
www.gluten.net

Gluten Free Diet
www.glutenfreediet.ca

Allergies

Kids with Food Allergies
www.kidswithfoodallergies.org

Canadian Society of Allergy and Clinical Immunology
http://csaci.ca/

Anaphylaxis Canada
http://www.anaphylaxis.ca/

Canadian Allergy, Asthma and Immunology Foundation
http://www.allergyfoundation.ca/

Asthma and Allergy Foundation of America
http://www.aafa.org/

Food Allergy Research and Education
http://www.foodallergy.org/

Asthma

The Asthma Society of Canada
www.asthma.ca

The Lung Association
http://www.lung.ca/diseases-maladies/asthma-asthme_e.php

Asthma Kids
www.asthmakids.ca

Asthma Society of Canada
www.asthma.ca

Asthma.com
www.asthma.com

Crohn's/Colitis

Crohn's and Colitis Foundation of America
http://www.ccfa.org/

Crohn's and Colitis UK
http://www.crohnsandcolitis. org.uk/Home

Crohn's and Colitis Canada
http://www.crohnsandcolitis.ca

Eosinophilic Disorders

American Partnership for Eosinophilic Disorders
www.apfed.org

Cincinnati Children's – Cincinnati Center for Eosinophilic Disorders
http://www.cincinnatichildrens. org/service/c/eosinophilic- disorders/default/

Children's Hospital of Philadelphia – Center for Pediatric Eosinophilic Disorders
http://www.chop.edu/service /center-for-pediatric- eosinophilic- disorders/home.html

Cured
http://curedfoundation.org/

Registry for Eosinophilic Gastrointestinal Disorders
http://regid.org/

Diabetes

University of Sydney Glycemic Index
http://www.glycemicindex.com/

American Diabetes Association
www.diabetes.org

Canadian Diabetes Association
www.diabetes.ca

IBS

Irritable Bowel Syndrome
Self Help and Support Group
www.ibsgroup.org

IBS Network
www.theibsnetwork.org

Eczema

The Eczema Society of Canada
http://www.eczemahelp.ca/

PKU

The Canadian PKU and
Allied Disorders
www.canpku.org

PKU News
www.pkunews.org

The National Society for
Phenylketonuria
www.nspku.org

Appendix

Here you will find some forms that you may find handy. I realize that this is a small book and there may not be enough room to write in them adequately, so all of these forms are available on my website (www.wholehealthoptions.ca) for you to download and customize if you like. They aren't fancy, they aren't complicated, but it's nice to get the information down and in one place, because it can be difficult to remember everything.

Personally, I have a binder at home (with a divider to separate my two kids) with these sheets in them. That way I can add sheets as I need them and it is convenient enough for me to carry around to appointments, etc. Feel free to download the forms and make them your own. Some people add clipart, add a column, and delete a row, whatever. The main point is to make them something you would like to use, and will use. You may think, "how am I ever going to forget the day of his surgery" but trust me, 10 years down the road it may be a little harder to remember...

Here is a list of forms to get you started on being proactive with your health:

- Diet and Symptom Diary
- 3 Day Food Intake Form
- Medical Team
- Other Members of my Team
- Allergy Symptom Diary

- Rx Allergies
- Food Allergies
- Environmental Allergies
- Procedures
- Current Rx List

There is also a Bristol Stool Chart in here. Many people who have food restrictive diseases/disorders also have problems with their bowels. This chart will help you clinically describe your bowel movements to your doctor rather than just saying, "I had the runs". There are also some information sheets for you to use as a reference for allergies and Celiac Disease. It seems that there are so many different ways to label food; hopefully this will make it a little easier for you to navigate that ingredient list. Here are those references for you:

- Bristol Stool Chart
- Sources of Egg
- Sources of Milk
- Sources of Peanut
- Sources of Tree Nuts
- Sources of Soy
- Sources of Wheat
- Sources of Gluten
- Glycemic Index/Load

Diet and Symptom Diary

	Sun	Mon	Tue	Wed	Thur	Fri	Sat
Food and Drink (note time)							
Pain Scale 0-10 (note time)							
Bowel Mvmnt (time, Bristol Stool Chart #)							

3 Day Food Intake

	Day 1	**Day 2**	**Day 3**
Breakfast			
Snack			
Lunch			
Snack			
Dinner			
Snack			

Medical Team

Physician	
Specialty	
Phone Number	
Email	
Address	
Notes	

Physician	
Specialty	
Phone Number	
Email	
Address	
Notes	

Medical Team

Physician	
Specialty	
Phone Number	
Email	
Address	
Notes	

Physician	
Specialty	
Phone Number	
Email	
Address	
Notes	

Other Members of My Team

Pharmacist	
Phone Number	
Email	
Address	
Notes	

Nutritionist	
Specialty	
Phone Number	
Email	
Address	
Notes	

Other Members of My Team

Name	
Specialty	
Phone Number	
Email	
Address	
Notes	

Name	
Specialty	
Phone Number	
Email	
Address	
Notes	

Other Members of My Team

Name	
Specialty	
Phone Number	
Email	
Address	
Notes	

Name	
Specialty	
Phone Number	
Email	
Address	
Notes	

Allergy Symptom Diary

	Sun	Mon	Tue	Wed	Thur	Fri	Sat
Food Drink (note time)							
Reaction (note time)							
Notes							

Rx Allergies

Name	
Reaction	
Action	
Notes	

Name	
Reaction	
Action	
Notes	

Name	
Reaction	
Action	
Notes	

Food Allergies

Name	
Reaction	
Action	
Notes	

Name	
Reaction	
Action	
Notes	

Name	
Reaction	
Action	
Notes	

Food Allergies

Name	
Reaction	
Action	
Notes	

Name	
Reaction	
Action	
Notes	

Name	
Reaction	
Action	
Notes	

Environmental Allergies

Name	
Reaction	
Action	
Notes	

Name	
Reaction	
Action	
Notes	

Name	
Reaction	
Action	
Notes	

Environmental Allergies

Name	
Reaction	
Action	
Notes	

Name	
Reaction	
Action	
Notes	

Name	
Reaction	
Action	
Notes	

Procedures

Procedure	
Date	
Reason	
Outcome	
Notes	

Procedure	
Date	
Reason	
Outcome	
Notes	

Procedures

Procedure	
Date	
Reason	
Outcome	
Notes	

Procedure	
Date	
Reason	
Outcome	
Notes	

Procedures

Procedure	
Date	
Reason	
Outcome	
Notes	

Procedure	
Date	
Reason	
Outcome	
Notes	

Rx List

Name	
Dosage	
Reason	
Start Date	
Contradictions	
Side Effects	
Notes	

Name	
Dosage	
Reason	
Start Date	
Contradictions	
Side Effects	
Notes	

Rx List

Name	
Dosage	
Reason	
Start Date	
Contradictions	
Side Effects	
Notes	

Name	
Dosage	
Reason	
Start Date	
Contradictions	
Side Effects	
Notes	

Bristol Stool Chart

Type 1		Separate hard lumps, like nuts (hard to pass)
Type 2		Sausage-shaped but lumpy
Type 3		Like a sausage but with cracks on its surface
Type 4		Like a sausage or snake, smooth and soft
Type 5		Soft blobs with clear-cut edges (passed easily)
Type 6		Fluffy pieces with ragged edges, a mushy stool
Type 7		Watery, no solid pieces. **Entirely Liquid**

(19)

Sources of Egg

Contain Egg

- Albumin
- Apovitellin
- Cholesterol free egg substitute (e.g. Eggbeaters®)
- Dried egg solids, dried egg
- Egg, egg white, egg yolk
- Egg wash
- Eggnog
- Fat substitutes
- Globulin
- Livetin
- Lysozyme
- Mayonnaise
- Meringue, meringue powder
- Ovalbumin
- Ovoglobulin
- Ovomucin
- Ovomucoid
- Ovotransferrin
- Ovovitelia
- Ovovitellin
- Powdered eggs
- Silici albuminate
- Simplesse
- Trailblazer
- Vitellin
- Whole egg

May Contain Egg

- Artificial flavoring
- Lecithin
- Natural flavoring
- Nougat

(20)

Sources of Milk

Contain Milk

- Butter [artificial butter, artificial butter flavor, butter, butter extract, butter fat, butter flavored oil, butter solids, dairy butter, natural butter, natural butter flavor, whipped butter]
- Casein & caseinates [ammonium caseinate, calcium caseinate, magnesium caseinate, potassium caseinate, sodium caseinate, hydrolyzed casein, iron caseinate, zinc caseinate]
- Cheese [cheese (all types), cheese flavor (artificial and natural), cheese food, cottage cheese, cream cheese, imitation cheese, vegetarian cheeses with casein]
- Cream, whipped cream
- Curds
- Custard
- Dairy product solids
- Galactose
- Ghee
- Half & Half
- Hydrolysates [casein hydrolysate, milk protein hydrolysate, protein hydrolysate, whey hydrolysate, whey protein hydrolysate]
- Ice cream, ice milk, sherbet
- Lactalbumin, lactalbumin phosphate
- Lactate solids
- Lactyc yeast
- Lactitol monohydrate
- Lactoglobulin
- Lactose

- Lactulose
- Milk [acidophilus milk, buttermilk, buttermilk blend, buttermilk solids, cultured milk, condensed milk, dried milk, dry milk solids (DMS), evaporated milk, fat-free milk, fully cream milk powder, goat's milk, Lactaid® milk, lactose-free milk, low-fat milk, malted milk, milk derivative, milk powder, milk protein, milk solids, milk solid pastes, non-fat dry milk, non-fat milk, non-fat milk solids, pasteurized milk, powdered milk, sheep's milk, skim milk, skim milk powder, sour milk, sour milk solids, sweet cream buttermilk powder, sweetened condensed milk, sweetened condensed skim milk, whole milk, 1% milk, 2% milk]
- Milk fat, anhydrous milk fat
- Nisin preparation
- Nougat
- Pudding
- Quark
- Recaldent
- Rennet, rennet casein
- Simplesse (fat replacer)
- Sour cream, sour cream solids, imitation sour cream
- Whey [acid whey, cured whey, delactosed whey, demineralized whey, hydrolyzed whey, powdered whey, reduced mineral whey, sweet dairy whey, whey, whey protein, whey protein concentrate, whey powder, whey solids]
- Yogurt (regular or frozen), yogurt powder

May Contain Milk

- Natural flavoring
- Flavoring
- Caramel flavoring
- High protein flour
- Lactic acid (usually not a problem)
- Lactic acid starter culture
- "Non-dairy" products may contain casein
- Rice cheese
- Soy cheese

(21)

Sources of Peanut

Contain Peanut

- Arachic oil
- Arachis
- Arachis hypogaea
- Artificial nuts
- Beer nuts
- Boiled peanuts
- Cold pressed, extruded, or expelled peanut oil
- Crushed nuts, crushed peanuts
- Dry roasted peanuts
- Earth nuts
- Goober peas
- Goobers
- Ground nuts, ground peanuts
- Hydrolyzed peanut protein
- Hypogaeic acid
- Mandelonas
- Mixed nuts
- Monkey nuts
- Nu nuts flavored nuts
- Nut pieces
- Nutmeat
- Peanuts, peanut butter, peanut butter chips, peanut butter morsels
- Peanut flour
- Peanut paste
- Peanuts sauce, peanut syrup
- Spanish peanuts
- Virginia peanuts

May Contain Peanuts

- Artificial flavoring
- Baked goods
- Candy
- Chili
- Ethnic foods: African, Asian, Chinese, Indian, Indonesian, Thai,
- Chocolate
- Crumb toppings
- Hydrolyzed plant protein
- Hydrolyzed vegetable protein
- Marzipan
- Mole sauce

Vietnamese, Mexican
- Fried foods
- Flavoring
- Graham cracker crust

(22)

- Natural flavoring
- Nougat

Sources of Tree Nuts

Common Tree Nut Names

- Almond
- Beechnut
- Brazil nut
- Bush nut
- Butternut
- Cashew
- Chestnut
- Coconut
- Filbert
- Ginko nut
- Hazelnut
- Hickory nut
- Lichee nut
- Macadamia nut
- Nangai nut
- Pecan
- Pine nut
- Pistachio
- Shea nut
- Walnut

Complete list of tree nut names, botanical names and derivative names for tree nuts

- Almond paste
- Anacardium nuts
- Anacardium occidentale (Anacardiaceae) [botanical name, Cashew]
- Artificial nuts
- Beech nut
- Canarium ovatum Engl. in A. DC. (Burseraceae) [botanical name, Pili nut]
- Caponata
- Carya illinoensis
- Brazil nut
- Bertholletia excelsa (Lecythidaceae) [botanical name, Brazil nut]
- Bush nut
- Butternut
- Butyrospermum Parkii [botanical name, Shea nut]
- Fagus spp. (Fagaceae) [botanical name, beech nut]
- Gianduja
- Ginko nut

- (Juglandaceae) [botanical name, Pecan]
- Carya spp. (Juglandaceae) [botanical name, Hickory nut]
- Cashew
- Castanea pumila (Fagaceae) [botanical name, Chinquapin]
- Castanea spp. (Fagaceae) [botanical name, Chestnut (Chinese, American, European, Seguin)]
- Chestnut (Chinese, American, European, Seguin)
- Chinquapin
- Coconut
- Cocos nucifera L. (Arecaceae (alt. Palmae)) [botanical name, Coconut]
- Corylus spp. (Betulaceae) [botanical name, Filbert/hazelnut]
- Filbert
- Macadamia spp. (Proteaceae) [botanical name, Macadamia nut/Bush nut]
- Mandelonas
- Marzipan
- Mashuga nuts
- Nangai nuts
- Ginkgo biloba L. (Ginkgoaceae) [botanical name, Ginko nut]
- Hazelnut
- Heartnut
- Hickory nut
- Indian nut
- Juglans cinerea (Juglandaceae) [botanical name, Butternut]
- Juglans spp. (Juglandaceae) [botanical name, Walnut, Butternut, Heartnut]
- Karite (shea nut)
- Lichee nut
- Litchi chinensis Sonn. Sapindaceae [botanical name, Lichee nut]
- Lychee nut
- Macadamia nut
- Nut pieces
- Pecan
- Pesto
- Pigñolia
- Pili nut
- Pine nut
- Pine nut (Indian, piñon, pinyon, pigndi, pigñolia, pignon nuts)
- Pinon nut
- Piñon or Piñon nut

- Natural and artificial flavoring
- Natural nut extract (for example, almond extract)
- Nougat
- Nu-Nuts®
- Nut butters (e.g., Almond butter, Hazelnut butter, Brazil nut butter, Macadamia nut butter, Pistachio nut butter, Shea nut butter, Karike butter, as well as other nut butters)
- Nut meal
- Nutella ®
- Nutmeat
- Nut oil (e.g., Walnut oil as well as other nut oils)
- Nut paste
- Walnut (English, Persian, Black, Japanese, California)
- Pinus spp. (Pineaceae) [botanical name, Pine nut/piñon nut]
- Pistachio
- Pistacia vera L. (Anacardiaceae) [botanical name, Pistachio]
- Pralines
- runus dulcis (Rosaceae) [bontanical name, almond]
- Shea nut
- Sheanut
- Vitellaria paradoxa C.F. Gaertn. (Sapotaceae) [botanical name, Shea nut]

May contain tree nuts

- Natural and Artificial flavoring
- Mortadella

(24)

158

Sources of Soy

Contain Soy

- Edamame (soybeans in pods)
- Hydrolyzed soy protein
- Kinnoko flour
- Kyodofu (freeze dried tofu)
- Miso
- Natto
- Okara (soy pulp)
- Shoyu sauce
- Soy albumin
- Soy bran
- Soy concentrate
- Soy fiber
- Soy flour
- Soy formula
- Soy grits
- Soy milk
- Soy miso
- Soy nuts
- Soy nut butter
- Soy protein, soy protein concentrate, soy protein isolate
- Soy sauce
- Soy sprouts
- Soya
- Soya Flour
- Soybeans
- Soybean granules
- Soybean curd
- Soybean flour
- Soy lecithin
- Soybean paste
- Supro
- Tamari
- Tempeh
- Teriyaki sauce
- Textured soy flour (TSF)
- Textured soy protein (TSP)
- Textured vegetable protein (TVP)
- Tofu
- Yakidofu
- Yuba (bean curd)

May Contain Soy:

- Artificial flavoring
- Natural flavoring

- Asian foods (e.g. Japanese, Chinese, Thai, etc.)
- Hydrolyzed plant protein
- Hydrolyzed vegetable protein (HVP)

- Vegetable broth
- Vegetable gum
- Vegetable starch

(25)

Sources of Wheat

Contain Wheat

- All purpose flour
- Bran
- Bread (any type made with flour)
- Bread flour
- Bromated flour
- Bulgur
- Cake flour
- Cereal extract
- Couscous
- Crackers, cracker meal
- Durum flour
- Enriched flour
- Farina
- Flour
- Fu
- Germ
- Gluten
- Graham flour
- High gluten flour
- High protein flour
- Wheat, wheat berries, wheat bran, wheat flour, wheat germ, wheat gluten, wheat grass, wheat malt, wheat starch, wheat sprouts
- Instant flour
- Malt, malt extract
- Matzo, Matzoh, Matzah, Matza, matsa, matso, Matzo meal, Matzoh meal, Matzah meal, Matza meal ,matsa meal, matso meal, matsah meal or matsoh meal
- Noodles
- Pasta
- Pastry flour
- Phosphated flour
- Plain flour
- Seitan
- Self-rising flour
- Soft wheat flour
- Steel ground flour
- Stone ground flour
- Tabbouleh
- Unbleached flour
- Vital gluten
- White flour
- Whole wheat berries
- Whole wheat bread
- Whole wheat flour

May Contain Wheat

- Artificial flavoring, natural flavoring
- Caramel color
- Dextrin
- Food starch
- Gelatinized starch
- Hydrolyzed vegetable protein (HVP)
- Maltodextrin
- Modified food starch
- Monosodium glutamate, MSG
- Oats (may be contaminated with wheat due to agricultural cultivation practices)

(26)

- Shoyu
- Soy Sauce
- Surimi
- Tamari
- Teriyaki Sauce
- Textured vegetable protein
- Vegetable gum
- Vegetable starch

Sources of Gluten

Contain Gluten

- Wheat
- Varieties and derivatives of wheat such as:

  - wheatberries
  - durum
  - emmer
  - semolina
  - spelt
  - farina
  - farro
  - graham
  - KAMUT® khorasan wheat
  - einkorn wheat

- Rye
- Barley
- Triticale
- Malt in various forms including: malted barley flour, malted milk or milkshakes, malt extract, malt syrup, malt flavoring, malt vinegar
- Brewer's Yeast

Common foods that contain gluten

- Pastas: raviolis, dumplings, couscous, and gnocchi
- Noodles: ramen, udon, soba (those made with only a percentage of buckwheat flour) chow mein, and egg noodles. (Note: rice noodles and mung bean noodles are gluten free)
- Breads and Pastries: croissants, pita, naan, bagels, flatbreads, cornbread, potato bread, muffins, donuts, rolls
- Crackers: pretzels, goldfish, graham crackers
- Baked Goods: cakes, cookies, pie crusts, brownies

- Cereal & Granola: corn flakes and rice puffs often contain malt extract/flavoring, granola often made with regular oats, not gluten-free oats
- Breakfast Foods: pancakes, waffles, french toast, crepes, and biscuits.
- Breading & Coating Mixes: panko breadcrumbs,
- Croutons: stuffings, dressings
- Sauces & Gravies (many use wheat flour as a thickener)
- traditional soy sauce, cream sauces made with a roux
- Flour tortillas
- Beer (unless explicitly gluten-free) and any malt beverages
- Brewer's Yeast
- Anything else that uses "wheat flour" as an ingredient

Foods that may contain gluten (must be verified):

- Energy bars/granola bars – some bars may contain wheat as an ingredient, and most use oats that are not gluten-free
- French fries – be careful of batter containing wheat flour or cross-contamination from fryers
- Potato chips – some potato chip seasonings may contain malt vinegar or wheat starch
- Processed lunch meats
- Candy and candy bars
- Soup – pay special attention to cream-based soups, which have flour as a thickener. Many soups also contain barley
- Multi-grain or "artisan" tortilla chips or tortillas that are not entirely corn-based may contain a wheat-based ingredient

- Salad dressings and marinades – may contain malt vinegar, soy sauce, flour starch or dextrin if found on a meat or poultry product could be from any grain, including wheat
- Brown rice syrup – may be made with barley enzymes
- Meat substitutes made with seitan (wheat gluten) such as vegetarian burgers, vegetarian sausage, imitation bacon, imitation seafood (Note: tofu is gluten-free, but be cautious of soy sauce marinades and cross-contamination when eating out, especially when the tofu is fried)
- Soy sauce (though tamari made without wheat is gluten-free)
- Self-basting poultry
- Pre-seasoned meats
- Cheesecake filling - some recipes include wheat flour
- Eggs served at restaurants – some restaurants put pancake batter in their scrambled eggs and omelets, but on their own, eggs are naturally gluten-free
- Distilled beverages and vinegars
- Most distilled alcoholic beverages and vinegars are gluten-free. These distilled products do not contain any harmful gluten peptides even if they are made from gluten-containing grains.

Other items that must be verified:

- lipstick, lipgloss, and lip balm because they are unintentionally ingested
- communion wafers
- herbal or nutritional supplements
- drugs and over-the-counter medications

- vitamins & mineral supplements
- play-dough: children may touch their mouths or eat after handling wheat-based play-dough. For a safer alternative, make homemade play-dough with gluten-free flour.

Places where cross-contact can occur:

- toasters used for both gluten-free and regular bread
- flour sifters
- deep fried foods cooked in oil shared with breaded products
- shared containers including improperly washed containers
- condiments such as butter, peanut butter, jam, mustard, and mayonnaise may become contaminated when utensils used on gluten-containing food are double-dipped
- wheat flour can stay airborne for many hours in a bakery (or at home) and contaminate exposed preparation surfaces and utensils or uncovered gluten-free products
- oats — cross-contact can occur in the field when oats are grown side-by-side with wheat, select only oats specifically labeled gluten-free)
- pizza — pizzerias that offer gluten-free crusts sometimes do not control for cross-contamination with their wheat-based doughs
- French fries
- non-certified baked goods e.g. "gluten-free" goods from otherwise gluten-containing bakeries
- bulk bins at grocery stores or co-ops

(23)

Glycemic Index and Load

Food	Glycemic index (glucose = 100)	Serving size (grams)	Glycemic load per serving
Bakery Products and Bread			
Banana cake, made with sugar	47	60	14
Banana cake, made without sugar	55	60	12
Sponge cake, plain	46	63	17
Vanilla cake made from packet mix with vanilla frosting (Betty Crocker)	42	111	24
Apple, made with sugar	44	60	13
Apple, made without sugar	48	60	9
Waffles, Aunt Jemima (Quaker Oats)	76	35	10
Bagel, white, frozen	72	70	25
Baguette, white, plain	95	30	15
Coarse barley bread, 75-80% kernels, average	34	30	7
Hamburger bun	61	30	9

Food	Glycemic index (glucose = 100)	Serving size (grams)	Glycemic load per serving
Kaiser roll	73	30	12
Pumpernickel bread	56	30	7
50% cracked wheat kernel bread	58	30	12
White wheat flour bread	71	30	10
Wonder™ bread, average	73	30	10
Whole wheat bread, average	71	30	9
100% Whole Grain™ bread (Natural Ovens)	51	30	7
Pita bread, white	68	30	10
Corn tortilla	52	50	12
Wheat tortilla	30	50	8
Beverages			
Coca Cola®, average	63	250 mL	16
Fanta®, orange soft drink	68	250 mL	23
Lucozade®, original (sparkling glucose drink)	95±10	250 mL	40
Apple juice, unsweetened, average	44	250 mL	30
Cranberry juice cocktail (Ocean	68	250 mL	24

Food	Glycemic index (glucose = 100)	Serving size (grams)	Glycemic load per serving
Spray®)			
Gatorade	78	250 mL	12
Orange juice, unsweetened	50	250 mL	12
Tomato juice, canned	38	250 mL	4
Breakfast Cereals and Related Products			
All-Bran™, average	55	30	12
Coco Pops™, average	77	30	20
Cornflakes™, average	93	30	23
Cream of Wheat™ (Nabisco)	66	250	17
Cream of Wheat™, Instant (Nabisco)	74	250	22
Grapenuts™, average	75	30	16
Muesli, average	66	30	16
Oatmeal, average	55	250	13
Instant oatmeal, average	83	250	30
Puffed wheat, average	80	30	17
Raisin Bran™	61	30	12

Food	Glycemic index (glucose = 100)	Serving size (grams)	Glycemic load per serving
(Kellogg's)			
Special K™ (Kellogg's)	69	30	14
Grains			
Pearled barley, average	28	150	12
Sweet corn on the cob, average	60	150	20
Couscous, average	65	150	9
Quinoa	53	150	13
White rice, average	89	150	43
Quick cooking white basmati	67	150	28
Brown rice, average	50	150	16
Converted, white rice (Uncle Ben's®)	38	150	14
Whole wheat kernels, average	30	50	11
Bulgur, average	48	150	12
Cookies and Crackers			
Graham crackers	74	25	14
Vanilla wafers	77	25	14
Shortbread	64	25	10
Rice cakes, average	82	25	17

Food	Glycemic index (glucose = 100)	Serving size (grams)	Glycemic load per serving
Rye crisps, average	64	25	11
Soda crackers	74	25	12
Dairy Products and Alternatives			
Ice cream, regular	57	50	6
Ice cream, premium	38	50	3
Milk, full fat	41	250mL	5
Milk, skim	32	250 mL	4
Reduced-fat yogurt with fruit, average	33	200	11
Fruits			
Apple, average	39	120	6
Banana, ripe	62	120	16
Dates, dried	42	60	18
Grapefruit	25	120	3
Grapes, average	59	120	11
Orange, average	40	120	4
Peach, average	42	120	5
Peach, canned in light syrup	40	120	5
Pear, average	38	120	4
Pear, canned in pear juice	43	120	5
Prunes, pitted	29	60	10

Food	Glycemic index (glucose = 100)	Serving size (grams)	Glycemic load per serving
Raisins	64	60	28
Watermelon	72	120	4
Beans and Nuts			
Baked beans, average	40	150	6
Blackeye peas, average	33	150	10
Black beans	30	150	7
Chickpeas, average	10	150	3
Chickpeas, canned in brine	38	150	9
Navy beans, average	31	150	9
Kidney beans, average	29	150	7
Lentils, average	29	150	5
Soy beans, average	15	150	1
Cashews, salted	27	50	3
Peanuts, average	7	50	0
Pasta and Noodles			
Fettucini, average	32	180	15
Macaroni, average	47	180	23
Macaroni and Cheese (Kraft)	64	180	32
Spaghetti, white, boiled, average	46	180	22

Food	Glycemic index (glucose = 100)	Serving size (grams)	Glycemic load per serving
Spaghetti, white, boiled 20 min, average	58	180	26
Spaghetti, wholemeal, boiled, average	42	180	17
Snack Foods			
Corn chips, plain, salted, average	42	50	11
Fruit Roll-Ups®	99	30	24
M & M's®, peanut	33	30	6
Microwave popcorn, plain, average	55	20	6
Potato chips, average	51	50	12
Pretzels, oven-baked	83	30	16
Snickers Bar®	51	60	18
Vegetables			
Green peas, average	51	80	4
Carrots, average	35	80	2
Parsnips	52	80	4
Baked russet potato, average	111	150	33
Boiled white potato, average	82	150	21
Instant mashed potato, average	87	150	17
Sweet potato,	70	150	22

Food	Glycemic index (glucose = 100)	Serving size (grams)	Glycemic load per serving
average			
Yam, average	54	150	20
Miscellaneous			
Hummus (chickpea salad dip)	6	30	0
Chicken nuggets, frozen, reheated in microwave oven 5 min	46	100	7
Pizza, plain baked dough, served with parmesan cheese and tomato sauce	80	100	22
Pizza, Super Supreme (Pizza Hut)	36	100	9
Honey, average	61	25	12

(37)

Emergency Procedures

I really hope that this section does not get used a lot – read it, learn it, memorize it – but I hope you don't need to use it. This goes over what the emergency procedures are for anaphylactic reactions (and how to use the various epinephrine auto injectors on the market) as well as asthma emergencies. This is incredibly valuable information that needs to be learned by anyone who is caring for a person with anaphylaxis or asthma. It is your responsibility to know this information inside and out. But like I said, I hope you never need to use it.

Emergency Protocol for Anaphylaxis

1 Give epinephrine auto-injector (e.g. EpiPen® or Twinject® or Allerject®) at the first sign of a known or suspected anaphylactic reaction.
2 Call 9-1-1 or local emergency medical services. Tell them someone is having a life-threatening allergic reaction.
3 Give a second dose of epinephrine in 5 to 15 minutes if the reaction continues or worsens.
4 Go to the nearest hospital immediately (ideally by ambulance), even if symptoms are mild or have stopped. The reaction could worsen or come back, even after proper treatment. Stay in the hospital for an appropriate period of observation as decided by the emergency department physician (generally about 4 hours).
5 Call emergency contact person (e.g. parent, guardian, spouse).

(28)

How do I use EpiPen®?

Remove the EpiPen® Auto-Injector from the carrier tube and follow these 2 simple steps:

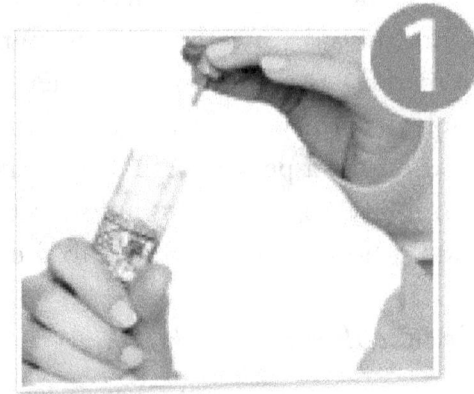

- Hold firmly with orange tip pointing downward.
- Remove blue safety cap by pulling straight up. Do not bend or twist.

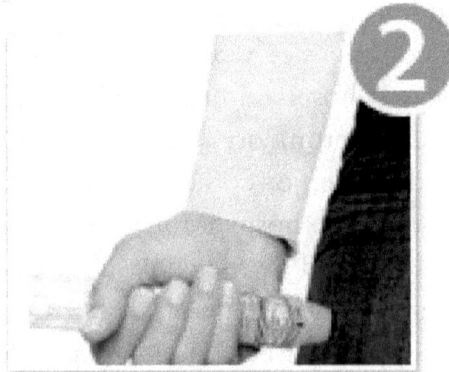

- Swing and push orange tip firmly into mid-outer thigh until you hear a "click."

- Hold on thigh for several seconds.

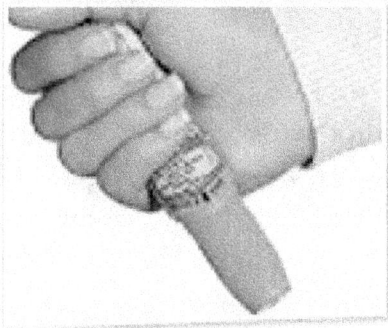

- When EpiPen® is removed the orange needle cover automatically extends to cover the injection needle, ensuring the needle is never exposed.

(29)

How do I use Twinject®?

Step 1 – Make sure your Twinject is ready

Examine your Twinject® 0.3 mg or Twinject® 0.15 mg regularly. It may not work if the medicine looks cloudy (has particles), pinkish, or more than slightly yellow, or if the expiration date has passed. In the event of a life-threatening allergic reaction, you should use an out of date product, if that is all you have. Do *not* remove the *green* caps until you are ready to use your Twinject®.

Step 2 – First dose

1   Pull off green end cap marked [1] to see a red tip. Never put thumb, finger or hand over the red tip.

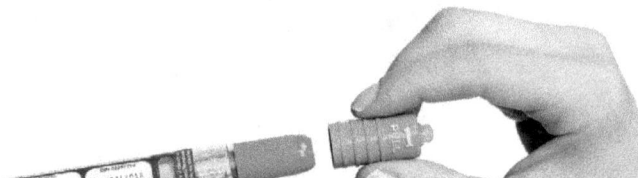

2   Pull of green end cap marked [2].

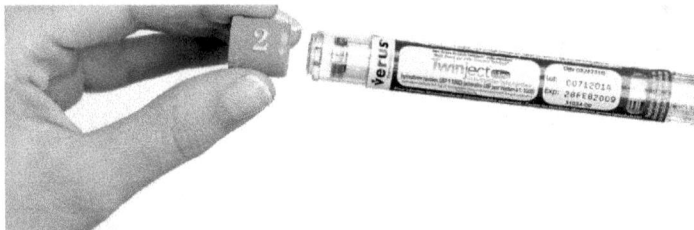

3   Place red tip against mid-thigh (injection can go through clothes).

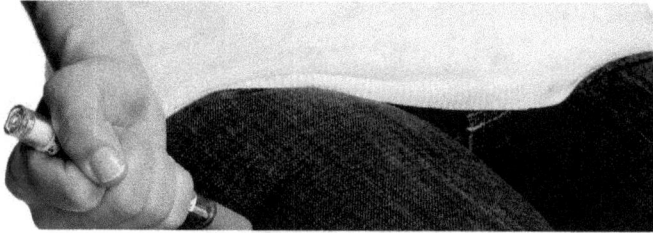

4   Press down hard until the needle enters your thigh through your skin – hold while slowly counting to 10.
5   Remove auto-injector and check red tip; if needle is exposed, you have received the dose.

    If not, repeat steps 3 and 4.

6   Call 911 or the closest emergency department as soon as you administer the first dose.

Step 3 – Prepare for the second dose

1   Unscrew and remove red tip. Beware of the exposed needle.
2   Holding blue hub at needle base, remove syringe from barrel.

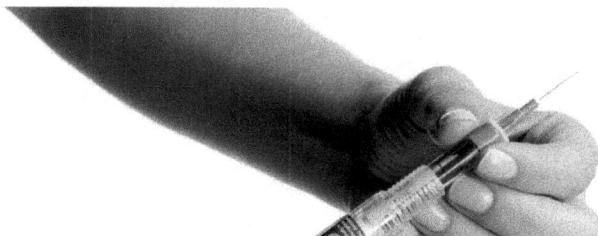

3   Slide yellow collar off plunger.

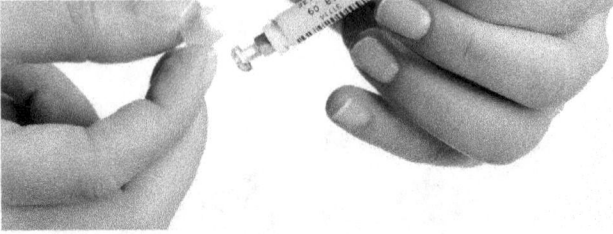

4   Pause here. If your symptoms have not improved within
     10 minutes since the first injection, proceed with steps 5
     and 6.
5   Put the needle into your thigh (upper leg).

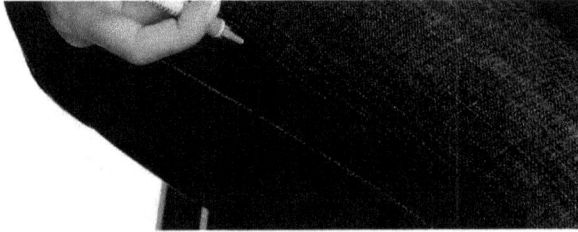

6   Push the plunger down all the way. Give the used
     Twinject® to a healthcare worker for proper disposal. Do
     not throw it away in the trash.

(30)

How do I use Allerject®

Allerject™ contains an electronic voice instruction system to help guide you through each step of your injection. If the voice instructions do not work for any reason, use Allerject™ as instructed in these Instructions for Use. It will still work during an allergic reaction emergency.

1   Pull Allerject™ from the outer case

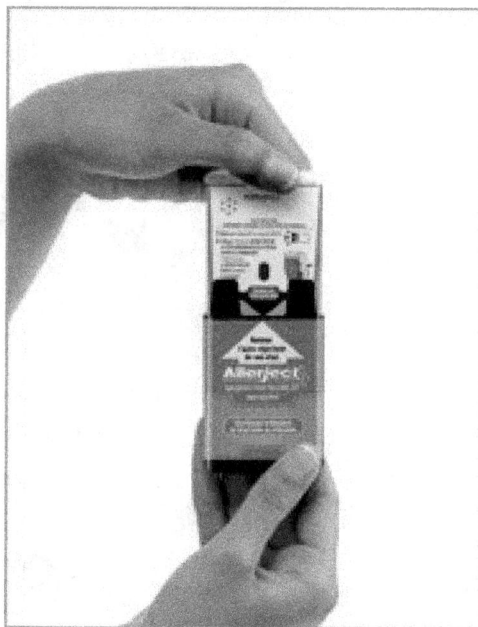

Do not go to step 2 until you are ready to use Allerject™. If you are not ready to use, put it back in the outer case.

2   Pull off red safety guard

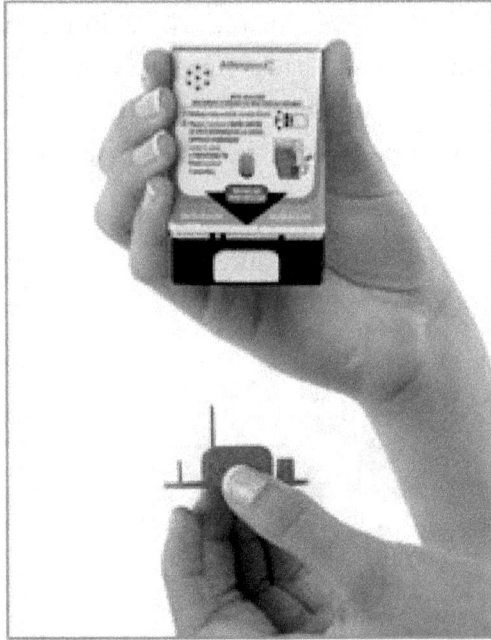

To reduce the chance of an accidental injection, do not touch the black base of the auto-injector, which is where the needle comes out. If an accidental injection happens, get medical help immediately.

NOTE: The safety guard is meant to be tight. Pull firmly to remove.

3   Place black end against the middle of the outer thigh
    (through clothing, if necessary), then press firmly and hold
    in place for five seconds.

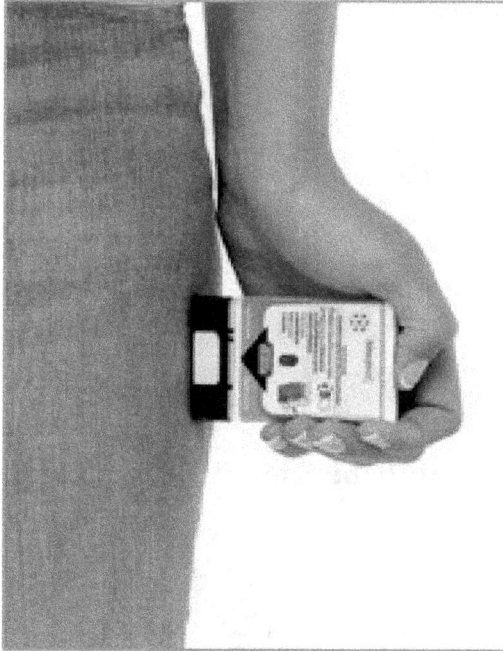

Only inject into the middle of the outer thigh (upper leg). Do
not inject into any other location.

Note: Allerject™ makes a distinct sound (click and hiss) when
you press it against your leg. This is normal and indicates
Allerject™ is working correctly.

4   Seek immediate medical or hospital care.
5   Replace the outer case and take your used Allerject™ with
    you to your pharmacist or physician for proper disposal and
    replacement.

(31)

Emergency Protocol for Asthma

Your aims during an asthma attack are to ease the breathing and if necessary get medical help.

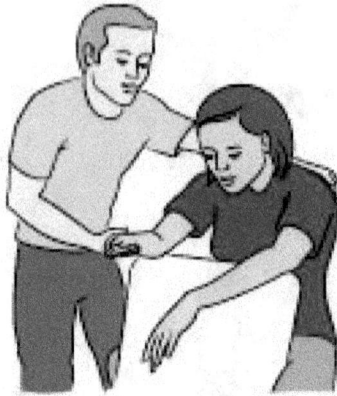

1   You need to keep the casualty calm and reassure them.

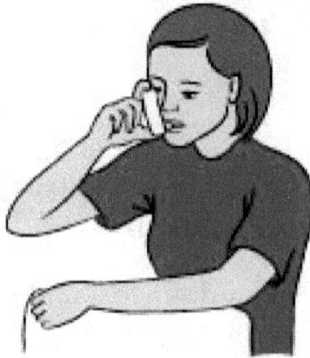

2   If they have a blue reliever inhaler then encourage them to use it. Children may have a spacer device and you should encourage them to use that with their inhaler also. It should relieve the attack within a few minutes.

3 Encourage the casualty to breathe slowly and deeply.

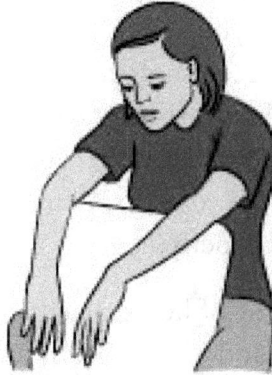

4 Encourage the casualty to sit in a position that they find most comfortable. Do not lie the casualty down.
5 Mild asthma attack should ease within a few minutes of them using their inhaler. If it doesn't then assist them to use their inhaler (one or two puffs) every two minutes until they have had 10 puffs.
6 Monitor their vital signs - breathing, level of response and pulse.
7 Caution: If this is the first attack, the attack is severe, the inhaler has no effect or the attack appears to be getting worse, dial 911 for an ambulance.

(32)

Emergency Protocol for Hemorrhaging

While not common, if you suffer from any of the gastrointestinal diseases/disorders discussed in this book, there may be a chance that you can hemorrhage severely from any portion of the gastrointestinal tract. Hemorrhage is a fancy term for bleeding, and it can lead to serious consequences if not recognized and/or treated properly.

If you notice these signs of hemorrhaging, contact your doctor. If the amount of the blood is significant, then go directly to the emergency department.

- Bright red stool (indicates a lower GI bleed)
- Black stool (indicates an upper GI bleed, or a slow bleed)
- Weakness
- Fatigue
- Blood in your vomit (indicates an upper GI bleed)
- Shortness of breath
- Paleness

(33)

Acknowledgements

First of all, I want to thank my entire family, immediate and extended. Each and every one of you played a part in helping me get this book out there. Whether it was just being part of my life and making me who I am today, reading excerpts from this book, or providing me with experiences that helped me write this book – thank you. A real big thank you to my kids and hubby!

Secondly, to all the doctors, nurses, specialists, social workers, and EMT's that have worked with me and my family over the years, thank you. I especially want to thank my childrens' current team because you all allowed me to have faith in other people caring for my kids and taught me how important it is to have a great relationship with your medical team. You are truly instrumental in keeping my kids healthy, my sanity in check, and me on my toes. Dr. J. D. Butzner, Dr. N. Cooper, Lisa Powell, Julia Wood, and Francine Abma-Vink – you all deserve an extra shout out!

Finally, I would like to thank Linda Ellis Eastman. Without your belief and confidence in me, before I even had it, I would not have been presented with this opportunity. Thank you for giving me that nudge into the water to see if I would sink or swim. Let's see if I can swim that marathon now!

(18)

About the Author

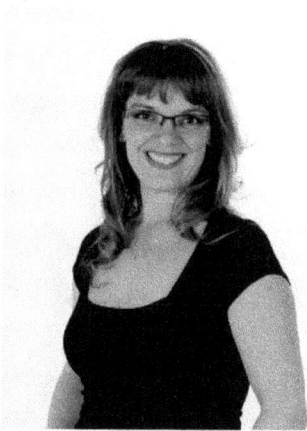

Throughout Brandy's life, she has been thrown into various health issues personally and with loved ones that has instilled a need for knowledge to help her to understand what was happening and learn more in an effort to help anyone who may need it. In addition to that, she and her children have a rare disorder that drastically restricts the food that they can eat, and over the years that led her to figure out how foods can not only nourish a body, but help it. This drove her to learn more formally.

Brandy holds a Bachelor of Arts degree with a double major in English and Sociology from the University of Lethbridge, as well as a Nutritional Consulting Practitioner Diploma (Honors) and a Certificate in Sports and Fitness Nutrition (Honors) from the Alive Academy. This education has provided her with the theoretical knowledge that she has always known instinctively and has always been passionate about. With this background, Brandy founded Whole Health Options and has been able to reach out and help many more people.

Brandy specializes in helping people who need to restrict their foods due to certain disease/disorders they may have, but she also enjoys the challenge that each and every client provides her regardless of their current situation. Her philosophy is simple; health and happiness can be achieved as long as you approach it with an open heart and mind. You can learn more about Brandy and the work she does by visiting:

Whole Health Options

www.wholehealthoptions.ca

bgassner@wholehealthoptions.ca

References

1 Medicinenet.com, 2014. [Online]. Available: http://www.medicinenet.com. [Accessed: 04- Aug- 2014].

2 Magazine, 'Let everyone eat bread :: Summer 2013 :: Washington State Magazine', *Wsm.wsu.edu*, 2014. [Online]. Available: http://wsm.wsu.edu/s/index.php?id=1031. [Accessed: 04- Aug- 2014].

3 Northwestern.edu, 'Northwestern University', 2014. [Online]. Available: http://northwestern.edu. [Accessed: 14- Apr- 2014].

4 Info.dhcla.com, 2015. [Online]. Available: http://info.dhcla.com/Portals/219289/images/inflammatory %20bowel%20disease-%20crohn%27s%20and%20ulcerative %20colitis.jpg. [Accessed: 01- Feb- 2015].

5 Webmd.com, 'Diverticula', 2014. [Online]. Available: http://www.webmd.com/digestive-disorders/diverticula. [Accessed: 07- May- 2014].

6 Uspharmacist.com, 'USPharmacist.com > Eosinophilic Esophagitis: A New Disease', 2014. [Online]. Available: http://www.uspharmacist.com/content/d/featured_articles/c /24726/. [Accessed: 01- May- 2014].

7 Allergyhome.org, 2014. [Online]. Available: http://www.allergyhome.org/handbook/files/2013/05/Signs _Symptoms-of-Anaphylaxis-685x412px.jpg. [Accessed: 02- Apr- 2014].

8   Gi.jhsps.org, 'Irritable Bowel Syndrome (IBS): Â Â Â Â
     Introduction', 2014. [Online]. Available:
     https://gi.jhsps.org/GDL_Disease.aspx?CurrentUDV=31&G
     DL_Cat_ID=024CC2E1-2AEB-4D50-9E02-C79825C9F9
     BF&GDL_Disease_ID=F5E21D6B-A88E-44F9-900F-7E295
     C50D38B. [Accessed: 04- Aug- 2014].

9   Homepage.eircom.net, 2014. [Online]. Available:
     http://homepage.eircom.net/~homeeconomics/proteins.htm.
     [Accessed: 27- Apr- 2014].

10   Depts.washington.edu, 'PKU Clinic - University of
     Washington, Seattle', 2014. [Online]. Available:
     http://depts.washington.edu/pku/about/diet.html.
     [Accessed: 30- Apr- 2014].

11   Asthma.ca, 'What is Asthma? - About Asthma - The Asthma
     Society of Canada', 2014. [Online]. Available:
     http://www.asthma.ca/adults/about/whatIsAsthma.php.
     [Accessed: 06- May- 2014].

12   Ellies-whole-grains.com, 2014. [Online]. Available:
     http://www.ellies-whole-grains.com/images/
     constipation.jpg. [Accessed: 09- May- 2014].

13   STACK, 'How to Assess Your Hydration Status', 2014.
     [Online]. Available:
     http://basketball.stack.com/nutrition/hydration/how-to-
     assess-your-hydration-status/. [Accessed: 17- May- 2014].

14   Webmd.com, 'Diarrhea Causes: Infection, IBS, Colitis, &
     More', 2014. [Online]. Available:
     http://www.webmd.com/digestive-disorders/understanding-
     diarrhea-basics. [Accessed: 24- May- 2014].

15   Acadiahealthclinic.com, 2014. [Online]. Available:
     http://acadiahealthclinic.com/wp-content/uploads/2014/04/
     eczema-prevention-tips.jpg. [Accessed: 02- Jun- 2014].

16 Med-health.net, 2014. [Online]. Available: http://www.med-health.net/images/10437462/image001.jpg. [Accessed: 10-Jun- 2014].

17 Balch, *Prescription for nutritional healing*, 1st ed. New York: Avery, 2006.

18 Turningpoint6.org, 2014. [Online]. Available: http://turningpoint6.org/wp-content/uploads/2014/05/Thank-You.jpg. [Accessed: 05- Aug- 2014].

19 Continence.org.au, 2014. [Online]. Available: http://www.continence.org.au/data/images/bristol_stool_chart.gif. [Accessed: 04- Aug- 2014].

20 Kidswithfoodallergies.org, 'Egg Allergy | How to Read a Label for Hidden Egg Names', 2014. [Online]. Available: http://www.kidswithfoodallergies.org/resourcespre.php?id=36&title=Egg_allergy_avoidance_list. [Accessed: 03- Aug- 2014].

21 Kidswithfoodallergies.org, 'Milk Allergy | How to Read a Label for Hidden Milk', 2014. [Online]. Available: http://www.kidswithfoodallergies.org/resourcespre.php?id=37. [Accessed: 03- Aug- 2014].

22 Kidswithfoodallergies.org, 'Peanut Allergy | How to Read a Label for Hidden Peanuts', 2014. [Online]. Available: http://www.kidswithfoodallergies.org/resourcespre.php?id=62&title=Peanut_allergy_avoidance_list. [Accessed: 03- Aug- 2014].

23 Celiac Disease Foundation, 'Sources of Gluten - Celiac Disease Foundation', 2013. [Online]. Available: http://celiac.org/live-gluten-free/gluten-free-diet/sources-of-gluten/. [Accessed: 03- Aug- 2014].

24 Kidswithfoodallergies.org, 'Tree nut allergy? Complete avoidance list for tree nuts', 2014. [Online]. Available: http://www.kidswithfoodallergies.org/resourcespre.php?id=6 0&title=Tree_nut_allergy_avoidance_list#sthash.QlV7W1yK .dpuf. [Accessed: 15- Aug- 2014].

25 Kidswithfoodallergies.org, 'Soy Allergy | How to Read a Label for Hidden Soy', 2014. [Online]. Available: http://www.kidswithfoodallergies.org/resourcespre.php?id=51 &title=Soy_allergy_avoidance_list. [Accessed: 15- Aug- 2014].

26 Kidswithfoodallergies.org, 'Wheat Allergy | How to Read a Label for Hidden Wheat', 2014. [Online]. Available: http://www.kidswithfoodallergies.org/resourcespre.php?id=5 2&title=Wheat_allergy_avoidance_list#sthash.LRLlzopl.dpuf. [Accessed: 15- Aug- 2014].

27 Images.medicinenet.com, 2014. [Online]. Available: http://images.medicinenet.com/images/illustrations/gastroes ophageal_reflux.jpg. [Accessed: 16- Aug- 2014].

28 Anaphylaxis Canada, 'Emergency Management of Anaphylaxis', 2014. [Online]. Available: http://www.anaphylaxis.ca/files/emergency%20management %20of%20anaphylaxis.pdf. [Accessed: 03- Sep- 2014].

29 Epipen.ca, 'How to use EpiPen', 2014. [Online]. Available: http://www.epipen.ca/en/about-epipen/how-to-use-epipen. [Accessed: 03- Sep- 2014].

30 Twinject.ca, 'How to use Twinject auto-injector to treat anaphylaxis', 2014. [Online]. Available: http://www.twinject.ca/how.php?lang=en. [Accessed: 03- Sep- 2014].

31 Sanofi | Allerject, 'Sanofi | Allerject', 2014. [Online]. Available: http://www.allerject.ca/en/epinephrine-autoinjector. [Accessed: 03- Sep- 2014].

32 www.sja.org.uk, 'Asthma', 2014. [Online]. Available: http://www.sja.org.uk/sja/first-aid-advice/breathing-problems/asthma.aspx. [Accessed: 03- Sep- 2014].

33 John P. Cunha, 'Gastrointestinal Bleeding Causes, Symptoms, Treatment - Gastrointestinal Bleeding Symptoms - eMedicineHealth', *eMedicineHealth*, 2014. [Online]. Available: http://www.emedicinehealth.com/gastrointestinal_bleeding/page3_em.htm. [Accessed: 04- Sep- 2014].

34 Webmd.com, 'Acid Reflux Disease Symptoms, Causes, Tests, and Treatments', 2014. [Online]. Available: http://www.webmd.com/heartburn-gerd/guide/what-is-acid-reflux-disease. [Accessed: 04- Sep- 2014].

35 Webmd.com, 'Heartburn Slideshow: Heartburn Causes, Triggers, and Remedies', 2014. [Online]. Available: http://www.webmd.com/heartburn-gerd/ss/slideshow-heartburn-overview. [Accessed: 04- Sep- 2014].

36 McGuire and K. Beerman, *Nutritional Sciences*, 1st ed. Belmont, Calif.: Thomson/Wadsworth, 2006, pp. 378-380; 437; 517; 520; 524; 526; 528; 530; 531.

37 Health.harvard.edu, 'Glycemic index and glycemic load for 100+ foods - Harvard Health Publications', 2014. [Online]. Available: http://www.health.harvard.edu/newsweek/Glycemic_index_and_glycemic_load_for_100_foods.htm. [Accessed: 06- Sep- 2014].

38 Brown, *Nutrition through the life cycle*, 1st ed. Australia: Thomson/Wadsworth, 2008, pp. 448, 495.

Other Work by Brandy

THE POWER OF TRANSFORMATION: REINVENTING YOUR LIFE

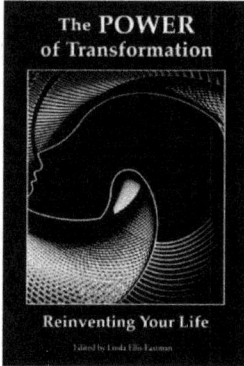

Anthology with 25 contributors, including Brandy

"Women are in constant transformation. Consider leaving home for college, beginning or ending a career, becoming a mother, empty nest syndrome, divorce, health challenges, and aging. Every woman globally faces personal or professional transformation at some point in her life. This book has been designed to provide you, the reader, with strategies and guidelines to help your transformation and personal reinvention move forward smoothly thus providing you with confidence, self-esteem and direction as you step into your next stage of life."

Linda Ellis Eastman

TAPPING INTO YOUR INNER VISION: TRANSFORMING YOUR LIFE & SHIFTING YOUR MIND

Anthology releasing 2015

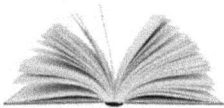

THE PROFESSIONAL WOMAN

Anthology releasing 2015

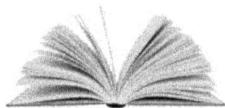

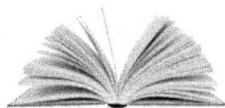

THE WOMAN'S BOOK OF EMPOWERMENT & CONFIDENCE: 356 DAILY AFFIRMATIONS VOLUME II

Releasing 2015